Hand Reflexology

Jürgen Kaiser,
Alexander Scharmann, M.D.,
and Beate Poyck-Scharmann, M.D.

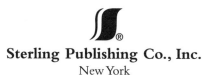

Sterling Publishing Co., Inc.
New York

The Authors

Jürgen Kaiser, the head of a large balneology department, is a certified massage therapist and balneologist. Since 1982, he has conducted intensive research into reflexology, rediscovering hand reflexology and developing a new therapeutic treatment called "neuroderm therapy." In 1993, he founded the Seminarzentrum Kaiser, a training center in Ofterschwang, Germany.

Beate Poyck-Scharmann, M.D., and Alexander Scharmann, M.D., have their own practice as general practitioners in Sonthofen, Germany. In addition, both specialize in sports medicine and naturopathy. Besides their teaching commitments, they are the medical consultants in charge at the Seminarzentrum Kaiser.

Library of Congress Cataloging-in-Publication Data Available

10 9 8 7 6 5 4 3 2

Published by Sterling Publishing Company, Inc.
387 Park Avenue South, New York, N.Y. 10016
First published in Austria under the title *Hand-Reflexzonen-Massage*
and © 1994 by Verlag Orac, a division of Verlag Kremayr & Sheriau, Vienna
English translation © 2000 by Sterling Publishing Company, Inc.
Distributed in Canada by Sterling Publishing
%Canadian Manda Group, One Atlantic Avenue, Suite 105
Toronto, Ontario, Canada M6K 3E7
Distributed in Great Britain and Europe by Cassell PLC
Wellington House, 125 Strand, London WC2R 0BB, England
Distributed in Australia by Capricorn Link (Australia) Pty Ltd.
P.O. Box 6651, Baulkham Hills, Business Centre, NSW 2153, Australia

Sterling ISBN 0-8069-5535-X

Contents

Preface

In our modern day and age, there is scarcely an area of life that has not been examined in terms of its relevance to health. In fact, we can hardly enjoy ourselves or have fun anymore without worrying about the consequences on our health.

Food, for example, should not simply be tasty—it must also be good for us. When we study the menu at a restaurant, we often worry about how much cholesterol and how many toxins, preservatives, and even viruses the different items may contain. Likewise, leisure-time sports are no longer just for recreation—they are expected to increase our fitness and stamina. We no longer go for a leisurely stroll—we do power walking instead. We go swimming and jogging and practice tai chi or qigong all for their health benefits.

Because we spend so much time in a sedentary position (in our cars, at the office, in front of the TV), the controversial question often arises as to what a "healthy" sitting posture looks like. There is also some debate regarding what constitutes "healthy" mattresses, "healthy" sleeping positions, and "healthy" sleep itself. Hardly anybody talks about comfort anymore—sleep has to be healthy first and foremost.

Shoes, clothes, hats, socks, underwear—everything has to comply with certain health standards. You will rarely find a car commercial these days that doesn't mention the health aspect, be it regarding the car's interior climate or the orthopedic car seats. And you can't enjoy sunbathing without being concerned about the adverse effects on your health; even the supposedly "healthy" sunblocks have come under scrutiny.

Of course, we could say, this is all just as well—doesn't it show that people have become more health-conscious and take better care of themselves than in the old days, when everybody was out to enjoy the pleasures of life and wasn't aware of how they could possibly endanger one's health? Yet an increased awareness of health-related issues often goes hand in hand with disillusionment over the capabilities of modern medicine. Today's health awareness is closely linked to the realization that physical and mental well-being can be achieved only with input and help from the individual. Self-help requires information from the media as well as a critical examination of the therapeutic measures recommended by the medical profession. And with both, patients are becoming increasingly more responsible for and involved in the decisions regarding their own treatment.

The topics discussed in this book—the theory and practice of hand reflexology—could make a significant contribution toward the development of modern-day patients. These are people who don't see dangers to their health everywhere, and who don't lose sight of the good things in life; yet, at the same time, they view health as a task that requires their continual attention. They don't just complain about the blows that fate has dealt them, but actively try to cope in the best way they can with whatever life throws in their direction.

Dr. Hans Hermann von Wimpffen, Editor

Introduction

Alternative Healing Methods and Conventional Medicine

What Is Health?

Thanks to sophisticated examination methods and modern technology, today diseases can be recognized at the start and highly effective medicines allow for successful treatment. However, this does not automatically result in a state of overall health. It is very difficult to define the term "health." Medical science can only provide guidelines in the form of values that can be measured and compared, such as blood counts, ECGs, or pulmonary function. But health also encompasses areas such as personal feelings, social circumstances, and environmental influences. Health could be described as a state of complete physical and mental well-being, for which there are no standardized values; therefore, evaluation remains up to the individual.

On the Lookout for Additional Therapies

Modern medicine concentrates almost exclusively on what can be measured and presented by a machine. This makes it possible for many diseases to be recognized and treated, but does not achieve complete health. Therefore, more and more people today are looking for additional therapies to attain this state. Another important factor is the growing need for more personal treatment. Even though society in the industrialized world is basically progressive, open, and tolerant, individuals are likely to become increasingly lonely as the psychological and social ties of the family break down. This is reflected in an increase of ailments that are not primarily caused by a diseased organ. Instead, the symptoms result from a disturbed inner balance. These disorders are referred to as functional, psycho-vegetative, or psychosomatic conditions.

The Problem of "Pain"

Pain is one of the major symptoms for disorders of the type described above. In today's industrialized society, the way people cope with pain has become problematic.

Normally, pain indicates some sort of danger or serious dysfunction. It therefore acts as an important signal that is not only apparent to the affected person but also to the people in his or her surroundings. If a person is discontent in some way or feels tension in certain relationships, he or she will experience pain in a different way. Pain can act as a relief mechanism to get rid of tension, but it also becomes a signal designed to attract attention from the environment. This mechanism can become so out of control that the person develops actual physical disorders and noticeable symptoms of disease.

What Are "Alternative Therapies"?

With the above type of disorder, medicine and machines can alleviate only symptoms, so the causes of the suffering remain. This explains the despair and the discontent with which many people turn to the so-called alternative therapies. But what exactly are they? The boundaries between conventional medicine and alternative therapies aren't always clear-cut. Many alternative therapies were developed on the basis of experience and cannot always be proven scientifically in every respect. In addition, conventional medicine, meaning the medical methods that are scientifically recognized at a given time, is subject to constant change. The term "alternative therapies" is somewhat misleading in itself, as it suggests that these therapies could replace conventional treatment, which they usually cannot do.

So Far and Yet So Close

Another reason why people turn to alternative methods, which tend to have a strong philosophical link, is their need to make sense of their own existence. The concept of health having to do with the unity of body and soul has existed for a long time; it can be found whenever medical teaching is based on a certain philosophy. Yet many people today who follow the trend toward Eastern philosophy forget that Western philosophy also acknowledges the idea of body and soul in harmony, influenced by a superior cosmos. The symbolism of yin and yang aptly depicts a dynamic unit combining two opposite aspects. However, the idea of life in flux among contrasting influences is not unique to Eastern philosophy, as it can be found in the philosophies of almost all cultures.

Progress and Tradition

Modern medicine has enabled us to treat many life-threatening illnesses more successfully. Modern antibiotics combat serious infectious diseases. Intensive treatment combining medication and technology has improved the survival rate for people with serious injuries or life-threatening functional disorders of the body. The infant mortality rate has been lowered significantly, and many people today live to a ripe old age. Of course, nobody wants to do without these positive developments. Conventional medicine also enjoys a long and continuous tradition. The knowledge of the human body and its various functions is based on exact scientific research, which must always be considered when working in medicine.

Uses and Risks

Recently, serious, often bitter discussion has centered around the uses and the risks of conventional therapies, and there has been a greatly increased demand for alternative therapies with fewer side effects. However, if one judges conventional medicine critically, one has to be even more critical of alternative healing methods. If an alternative method goes against the foundations of modern medicine, it should be approached with extreme care, and even more so if its practitioners think they can treat illnesses without having sound medical knowledge. Should an alternative healing method be practiced by an unqualified therapist who may have given the wrong diagnosis, the patient could be gravely endangered.

Decisions, Decisions . . .

When choosing the appropriate therapy, an exact diagnosis is the most important consideration. Furthermore, the risks and the uses of the therapies in question should be evaluated carefully. Several factors play a role in this process:
- Known effects and side effects
- Therapist's ability to use this particular method
- Patient's willingness to be treated by this method
- Patient's physical and mental states
- Period of time available for the treatment

With all forms of therapy, it is important to make decisions and adhere to the chosen path. Both the therapist and the patient need to observe the treatment carefully, and they should also be willing to make changes in the therapy if this becomes necessary. It is therefore crucial for the relationship between the therapist and the patient to be based on honesty and trust.

United, Not Separate

Once all the above points have been addressed, it will no longer be an issue of conventional medicine versus alternative therapies. The key to optimal treatment and the path to a possibly more complete state of health can be found in combining conventional medicine and alternative therapies.

Together with Jürgen Kaiser, who developed the method of hand reflexology, we have built bridges in this book between alternative therapies and conventional medicine. In order for you to be able to walk securely on these bridges, we have provided solid guidelines so that even if you aren't well versed in medicine you can still apply the methods of hand reflexology successfully and safely. Clinical pictures detailing distinctive features and risks are also supplied, but we would nevertheless urge you to consult a physician in any instances of doubt.

The Aims of This Book

The design and the functions of the human body are fascinating subjects indeed, and in a time when many people have a disturbed relationship with their bodies, knowledge of one's body forms an important part of health education. Becoming familiar with certain clinical pictures doesn't mean that we are searching for signs of ill health. This should, in fact, show us the way to recovery or to maintaining good health. This book looks into a number of different clinical pictures that, in the experience of reflexologists, have responded well to this type of therapy. The recommended therapies apart from reflexology are examples only and are intended to help you understand their place in possible treatment. The use of medication often requires the knowledge of a specialist and should take place only in cooperation with a doctor whom you trust.

The History of Hand Reflexology

During the age of the Mayas and the Incas, the medicine men of these highly civilized cultures did not have any technical aids to help them diagnose and treat illnesses. It was then that reflexology was developed, providing a means of complex treatment and good diagnosis. The Mayas documented their findings for future generations by carving them into sacred stone plaques. When the Mayan civilization came to an end, these discoveries disappeared with it.

At the height of the Mayan civilization, from A.D. 300 to 700, great intellectual feats were achieved. Science was at the service of religion, and the Mayas specialized in three sciences: mathematics, astronomy, and medicine.

Mayan writing reached a higher standard than other systems of writing by Native Americans. Similar to Egyptian hieroglyphics, it combines ideographic and phonetic characters, and, to this day, has not been deciphered completely. Stone columns and plates were erected in honor of deities and rulers, and they were carved with inscriptions carrying a date.

In mathematics, the Mayas had discovered a system of constants that enabled them to develop their famous calendar. In order to determine the exact length of a sun year, exact astronomic measurements and observations of the stars were necessary. The orbits of the sun, the moon, and of Venus were discovered in this manner.

Yet everything the Mayas did ranked after their religion and mythology. Mayan mythology, for example, regards the planet Venus as a double of the king of Tula, who is also a god. Venus's role is to represent a movement that, after a

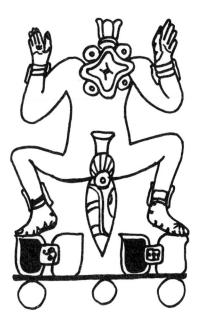

Figure 1

time in the depths of the earth, leads back to the realm of the sun. Figure 1, above, depicts the planet Venus setting in the evening.

In this picture, the hands and the feet are dominant and express movement. Hands and feet help to overcome an abyss (disease) to achieve happiness (health). The planet Venus represents love and harmony. This picture shows the importance of hand and foot reflexology.

The Mayas were well versed in the field of medicine. Excavations have brought forth skulls from which pieces of bone had been chiseled out. This indicates that, even in those days, skull surgery took place, most likely for religious reasons.

In 1938, Dr. Fitzgerald and Eunice Ingham, from America, discovered stone plaques that referred to foot reflexology, decoded them, and put them into a medical context (see "Foot Reflexology according to the Mayan Tradition"). Other stone plaques detailed hand reflexology, but these had been eroded by wind and rain, so they couldn't be deciphered. As a result, only foot reflexology became known worldwide. Hand reflexology was widely discussed, but experts could not determine where the various reflex zones lay.

Jürgen Kaiser, a professional masseur and medical balneologist (balneology is the science of the therapeutic use of baths), had trained in foot reflexology. In 1983, he researched hand reflexology intensively, putting the various zones into a topographical order. From what he discovered, he came to the conclusion that hand reflexology, if used correctly, could achieve even better results than foot reflexology. He also found it easier to practice, thus making it easier for the layperson to learn. He saw that people who learned hand reflexology would be able to help themselves and others, without the use of medicines, in cases of acute or chronic pain.

Foot Reflexology according to the Mayan Tradition

The altar at Copan contains Mayan engravings that referred to foot reflexology as early as a thousand years ago. The symbols were encoded so that only medicine men could understand their meaning.

Opposite, you can see a complete rendering of the altar at Copan, furnished by an archeologist named Frederick Catherwood. The stone plaque shows the treatment of the most important organs and limbs, as well as general guidelines for enhancing overall well-being. The Mayas practiced reflexology from head to foot, so the individual pictures are arranged topographically from top to bottom. Because a detailed discussion of the individual symbols would go beyond the scope of this book, we will take a closer look at only the first three pictures (top row of the plaque, from left to right). They detail treatment of the back of the head, the face, and the ears.

The horizontal bars found in the individual symbols represent the respective area of the body. Three bars refer to the head, two bars to the neck and chest, and one bar refers to the stomach-and-pelvis area.

The small circles in the individual pictures have a double meaning. First, they describe the technique and the direction of the massage. In picture 5, for example, the cervical spine is massaged from top to bottom. Second, they are also points of reference for the head area, the neck-and-chest area, and the stomach-and-pelvis area. If there are three small circles in a picture, a connection is made to the head. Therefore, in picture 14, depicting the stomach and the duodenum, taking food by mouth establishes the connection with the head.

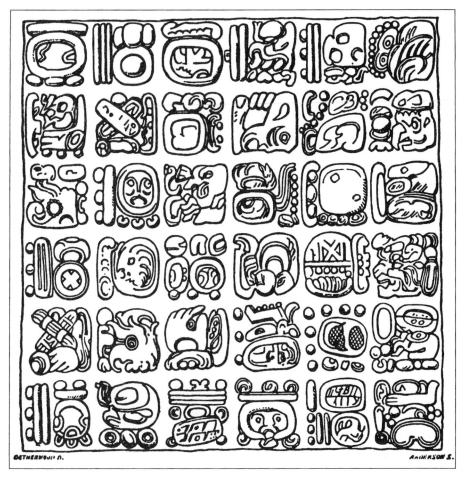

Rendering of the altar at Copan, provided by archeologist Frederick Catherwood

The individual pictures contain a great deal of coded information. What follows is a diagram interpreting the first three pictures on the Mayan plaque in relation to foot reflexology. The diagram shows the relationship of the foot reflex zones with the three pictures on the plaque.

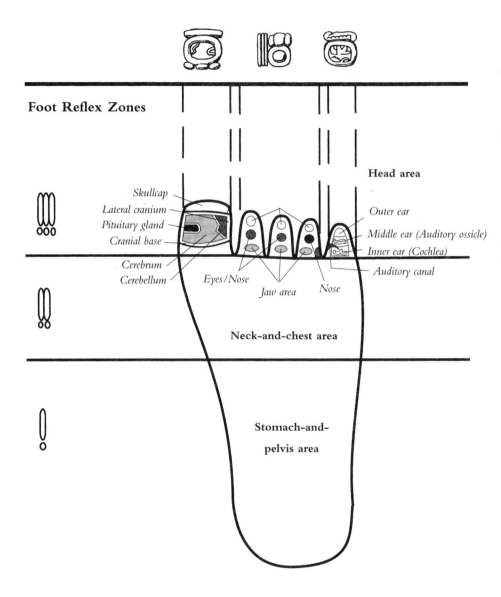

Foot Reflex Zones

Head area

Skullcap
Lateral cranium
Pituitary gland
Cranial base

Outer ear
Middle ear (Auditory ossicle)
Inner ear (Cochlea)
Auditory canal

Cerebrum
Cerebellum

Eyes/Nose

Jaw area

Nose

Neck-and-chest area

Stomach-and-pelvis area

Individual Symbols on the Mayan Plaque

Back of the Head

Top: Skullcap.
Middle: Entire skull, including the three areas of the brain.
Bottom: Shows the treatment of the big toes.

Face

Top: Second, third, and fourth toes.
Bottom: The small circle represents the face.
Left: The treatment is carried out from top to bottom; the three bars refer to the head area.

Ears

Top: Representation of the auditory ossicles.
Bottom: Circle representing the skull. At the top of the circle, the cochlea, at the bottom, the auditory canal.

Lymph Canals

Top: A canal system showing lymph flow.
Bottom: Toes and metacarpophalangeal toe joints.
Left: Points to the area of treatment between the toes. The two bars indicate the neck-and-chest area.

Cervical Spine

Top: A face distorted by pain.
Bottom: The seven cervical vertebrae, unordered.
Left: The small circles next to the toes indicate that the direction of the treatment should be from top to bottom.

Thoracic Spine

Left: The bronchial tubes are encircled by the 12 thoracic vertebrae.
Right and top: A lung.
Right and middle: A few ribs.
Right and bottom: Muscles of the chest.

Lumbar Spine, Sacrum, and Coccyx

Top: The five lumbar vertebrae, unordered.
Left: A half cross, representing the sacrum with the coccyx attached.
Right: The foot, including small circles indicating direction of treatment.

Shoulders and Arms

Left: Arms are crossed.
Right: Shoulder joint.
Bottom: Side of the body from the small toe up to the elbow.

Neck and Thyroid Gland

Top: Center of the thyroid gland, including the left and right thyroid lobes.
Left: Muscles belonging to the head.
Right: Position of the thyroid gland in the neck area.

Heart and Intercostal Muscles

Left: Dorsum of the foot at the height of the heart reflex zone, including the associated muscles.
Right: Massage point for the heart below the big toe on the ball of the foot.

Lungs, Windpipe, and Esophagus

Left: Esophagus (top) and windpipe (bottom), separated by the six thoracic vertebrae.
Right: Lung-superior and inferior lobes.

Heart-Related Zone

Left: Indicates that blood pressure is too high or too low.
Right: Poor blood circulation in the head area.

Diaphragm

Top: Separation of two parts of the body.
Bottom: The diaphragm has an important function. The crescent of the moon reflects the intake of air; the sun at the center of the picture stands for exhaling.

Stomach and Duodenum

Left: The vertical bar represents the beginning of the stomach area. The three small circles refer to the intake of food in the head-and-neck area.
Right: There is a connection between the stomach and the face. Below, a depiction of the duodenum.

Liver and Gallbladder

Left: Gallbladder duct (top) and pancreatic duct (bottom) meet.
Right: Liver, with adjoining gallbladder. The "tail" of the pancreas is wound around the liver.

Pancreas

Top: The "head" of the pancreas.
Bottom: The "body" of the pancreas.
Right: The "tail" of the pancreas, located at the level of the second lumbar vertebra.

Spleen

Left: Position of the spleen, level with the ninth thoracic vertebra.
Right: The spleen; the two small circles indicate that a change of function takes place with increasing age.
Bottom: For the massage, circular motions of varying directions are used.

Kidneys and Adrenal Glands

Top: Rear "wall" of the body.
Middle: Adrenal gland.
Bottom: Kidneys.

Ureter and Bladder

Left: The ureter runs from the kidneys downward.
Right: The prostate gland is depicted at the top; the circle containing the cross represents the bladder.

Small and Large Intestines

Left: Large intestine.
Right: The winding small intestine.

Lower Abdominal Organs

Left: Man with testicles, in side view, standing on two legs.
Right: Woman with head and long hair. The uterus is depicted inside the circle. She is shown in side view, kneeling on all fours.

Rectum and Anus

Left: Sphincter.
Right: Rectal cavity ending in the anus.

Abdominal and Pelvic Muscles

Left: The circle represents the entire abdominal area—the stomach at the top and the pelvis down below.
Right: The abdominal and pelvic muscles start just above the stomach and end level with the lower abdominal organs.

Hips

Left: Face of an old person.
Right: The ball-and-socket joint of the hip.

Legs

Top: Crossed legs, shown stronger than the arms.
Right: The foot is depicted at the bottom; pointing up from it is the Achilles tendon and its reflex zone.

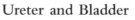

Knees

Left: The drawing portrays the entire leg, featuring a very large hip joint. The large protrusion at the center represents the knee.

Right: This shows the meniscus and the center of the joint.

Solar Plexus

Left: The foot shown features a notch between the first and second toes. Below these metacarpophalangeal toe joints, the reflex zone of the solar plexus can be found.

Right: The three or four vertically aligned small circles and the two horizontally aligned small circles can be used to determine the position of the solar plexus. Moving four pictures to the right and two pictures down takes us to picture 10, representing the heart. Moving two pictures to the right and three pictures down takes us to picture 14, the stomach. The solar plexus is located between the stomach and the heart.

Weight Reduction

Left: The three small circles connect pictures 2 (face), 5 (neck), 11 (esophagus), and 14 (stomach).

Top: Jaw cavity, including the tongue and the hard palate.

Bottom: Compressed stomach.

Stimulating the Sense of Taste

Center: Food intake is poor on the left side and good on the right.

Framework: The 10 small circles point toward the treatment zones. Each circle corresponds to a symbol on the plaque. The arms and heart do not receive treatment; this is indicated by circles 8 and 10 being crossed out.

Promoting Agility

Right: The drawing shows a person whose movements are restricted. It points to the spinal column and all joints.

Regulating Hormone Levels

Left: Neck area and thyroid gland.
Right: The pituitary gland is depicted at the top. The adrenal gland is represented in the top half of the circle, and the lower abdominal organs are shown below.

Increasing Endurance (Regulating Breathing)

Top: Working lung.
Bottom: Pointer toward the neck-and-chest area.

Restoring the Sense of Balance

Top: Points to picture 3 (ears) and the head area.
Middle: Head area (compressed).
Bottom: The body with all of its organs.

Improving General Well-being

Top: Points to picture 1 (head), focusing on the brain.
Bottom: Represents treatment of the whole body.

Increasing Sexual Potency

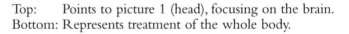

Top: Symbol of man, picture 1.
Bottom: Symbol of woman, picture 2. These figures point to picture 12 (heart-related zone, to increase blood pressure) and picture 21 (lower abdominal organs).

Calming Strokes Following the Structure of the Muscle

Top: Shows the hand performing calming strokes amid disorder.
Bottom: Glasses shape, conveying order and harmony.

Theoretical Foundations of Hand Reflexology

The Brain and the Nervous System

Wherever there are nerve endings, the entire body with its organs is represented. This includes the head, the skin, the feet, and the hands. These zones can be proven empirically, and have been used in the treatment of illnesses for thousands of years. In Asia, acupuncture was the prevalent therapy method; the Mayas and the Incas used reflexology. These kinds of therapy are gaining ever greater significance, as we can see from the fact that more and more traditional practitioners are using them and achieving good results.

Medical science has discovered that the reflex zones of the hand, the foot, and the head occupy the largest part of the cerebral cortex, and that impulses to these parts of the body can therefore travel a greater variety of routes and reach their destination far more often than for other parts of the body.

The somatosensory area of the cerebral cortex (on the left-hand side of the cross-section diagram in Figure 2) receives signals that the body's sensory organs send to the brain. The motor cortex (on the right-hand side) controls the body's movements. Because every part of the body corresponds to a specific segment on these cortexes, it is possible to project the whole body onto the surface of the brain. The individual parts of the body are represented in the motor cortex and the somatosensory cortex.

Figure 2

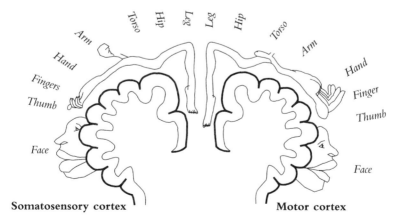

Reflexology has to incorporate the brain and the nervous system—probably the most amazing parts of the human body—in order to achieve good results. As with all other parts of the human body, the brain and the nervous system are composed of individual cells of which the components are known and can be examined separately. Nerve cells link up to form extremely complex networks, containing, it is estimated, more than a hundred billion nerve cells. A nerve cell usually receives information from hundreds, even thousands, of other nerve cells and transmits signals to just as many.

How Does Hand Reflexology Work?

With the following example, we can see how hand reflexology works. By applying pressure to the palm, using a circular motion, we trigger an energy impulse in the nerves surrounding the blood vessels (arteries and veins), of which the hand has many. By way of nerve tracts, the energy impulse reaches the spinal cord, where impulses are gathered. This collective energy potential travels along the nerve tracts that supply the various organs and body parts. An exchange of energy takes place in the body. Some of the energy flows to the brain; some of it flows to the respective organ or body part. If energy is distributed evenly, this means that the body is healthy. If there is no distribution of energy, all the energy flows back to where it came from, meaning the hand, and severe pain is felt in the part of the hand being massaged. This indicates that the corresponding organ or body part is in a state of weakness.

If the massage continues over a period of time, the collective energy potential in the spinal cord becomes so great that the barrier blocking the energy impulse breaks down from the pressure. Thus, energy can be distributed normally again, restoring harmony in the body.

An Example from Nature

To illustrate the above concept, it may help to picture the nervous system as a river with three branches (see Figure 3). One branch originates at the source of the river, which represents the hand. The second branch flows into a lake, representing an organ. The third branch ends in a water reservoir, symbolizing the brain. The water arrives in the reservoir and from there is distributed back into the three branches of the river.

The source (hand) brings forth water that travels unhindered along river-branch 1 to where the three river branches cross. The water travels the path of least resistance. Some of it flows along branch 2 to be absorbed completely by the lake (organ); the remainder flows along branch 3 and is collected in the reservoir (brain). If branch 3 becomes empty, the water from the reservoir is sent

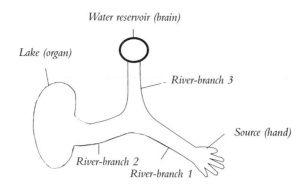

Water reservoir (brain)

Lake (organ)

River-branch 3

Source (hand)

River-branch 2

River-branch 1

Figure 3

back to the intersection of the river branches. Here, the stream divides, and some of the water flows into the lake, some of it back to the source. This means that less water is returning to the source than originated from it, and therefore water circulation is intact (see Figure 4). The analogy illustrates a healthy body in which the distribution of energy is functioning smoothly.

Figure 4

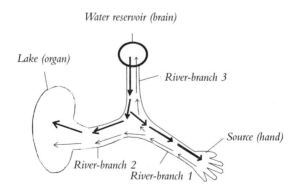

Water reservoir (brain)

Lake (organ)

River-branch 3

Source (hand)

River-branch 2

River-branch 1

If an organ is diseased or weakened, water circulation will appear as illustrated in Figure 5. In river-branch 2, a dam has been built. Thus, for any water gushing from the source (hand), the way to the lake (organ) has been blocked. The water travels to the water reservoir (brain) and from there straight back to the source (hand), causing flooding at the source. The water cycle has broken down.

This indicates that pain is felt in the respective reflex zone of the hand. The cause of this pain can be found in the corresponding organ.

Figure 5

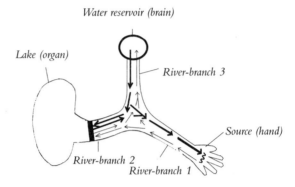

Water reservoir (brain)

Lake (organ)

River-branch 3

Source (hand)

River-branch 2

River-branch 1

Here, hand reflexology works in the following manner: The flow of water from the source (hand) is increased, so more water enters river-branches 1 and 2. This increases water pressure on the dam. Eventually, at a certain pressure, the dam will collapse and open the way to the lake (organ). The water cycle has been repaired; returning to reflexology, this means that the diseased or weakened organ has been treated successfully and the body has become healthy again.

Continuing with this analogy, we should be aware that there is a difference between acute complaints, which occur suddenly, and chronic complaints, which have been around for a long time. With acute complaints, the dam is narrow and can be broken down fairly easily. With chronic complaints, the dam is strong, with deep foundations, and a great deal of effort is needed to break it down. This means that continuous treatment of at least one to four months is necessary to achieve a significant improvement.

What Does Hand Reflexology Achieve?

Hand reflexology tells us whether or not there is any damage to the body or its organs; in other words, it helps in establishing a diagnosis.

It also allows us to treat pain and causes of illness effectively, which means that you can treat all the conditions that are described in this book on your own.

Of course, there are limits to this kind of therapy. For instance, in the case of heart attacks, severe accidents, bleeding, cancer, serious infectious diseases, and vegetative disorders, it is crucial to consult your doctor as soon as possible in order to avoid any complications.

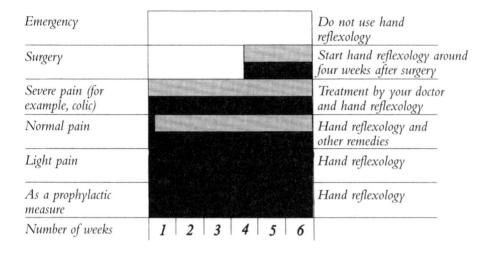

	1	2	3	4	5	6	
Emergency							Do not use hand reflexology
Surgery							Start hand reflexology around four weeks after surgery
Severe pain (for example, colic)							Treatment by your doctor and hand reflexology
Normal pain							Hand reflexology and other remedies
Light pain							Hand reflexology
As a prophylactic measure							Hand reflexology
Number of weeks	1	2	3	4	5	6	

 Hand reflexology   Treatment by doctor and alternative remedies   Do not use hand reflexology

The Different Zones

The various zones are identified on the basis of a diagram that is similar to the layout of a city on a map. The body corresponds to the city, and the hand is the map. The hand, as with a map, is divided up into horizontal and vertical zones (see Figure 6).

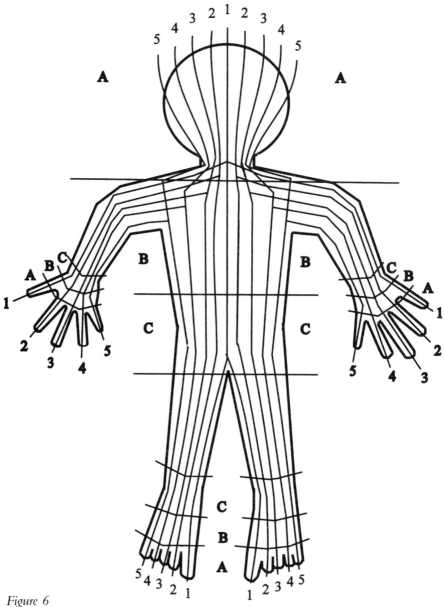

Figure 6

The first horizontal zone (A) comprises the head and neck, which correspond to the fingers and the metacarpophalangeal finger joints in the hand. The second horizontal zone (B) consists of the chest and upper stomach, which correspond to the metacarpus in the hand. The third horizontal zone (C) encompasses the stomach-and-pelvis region, which corresponds to the lower palm and the carpal bones in the hand. In addition, on the back of the hand, the carpal bones contain the zones for the region of the hip, leg, and knee.

The vertical zones are assigned to the fingers. The first zone runs along the thumb toward the center of the body. Zone 2 comprises the index finger, zone 3 the middle finger, zone 4 the ring finger, and zone 5 the little finger. The zones of the feet are similar.

Figure 7

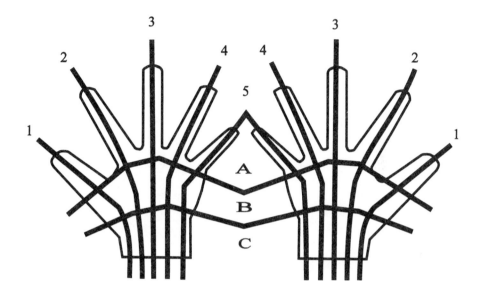

The Therapy

Of the five fingers on the hand, we choose the strongest one as our tool. This is the thumb, which stands in opposition to the four remaining fingers and has the most work to do. When it comes to treating a condition, you can choose the order in which you wish to massage the reflex zones on your hand. For diagnosing a condition, however, we suggest you follow the 10-step program described later in this chapter.

Position your thumb so that its tip touches the reflex zone you wish to treat, making sure that the thumbnail doesn't dig into the hand. Use a stationary, circular motion, and repeat it while simultaneously applying downward pressure. This releases an energy impulse that can have either a positive or a negative influence on the respective body part or organ.

For a positive influence, you need to build up energy. This is achieved by working in a circular motion toward the thumb of the hand you are treating; work clockwise on the right hand and counterclockwise on the left hand. This manner of treatment results in a buildup of energy.

For a negative influence, you need to conduct energy away from the respective organ or body part. This is achieved by working in a circular motion toward the little finger of the hand you are treating; work clockwise on the left hand and counterclockwise on the right hand (see Figure 8). This manner of treatment results in an energy drainage.

With each clinical picture in the following chapter, the table at the bottom of the page indicates the direction of the massage and the corresponding technique for either energy buildup or energy drainage. Massage the different zones according to the details given in the table.

Massaging should be continued until the pain experienced in the hand is reduced significantly. Depending on the condition, this can take between two and 10 minutes. If there is no significant improvement after 10 minutes, the treatment should be repeated every two to three hours. In the case of an acute complaint, as few as one to five sessions may suffice to reduce the pain. With chronic complaints, treatment needs to be carried out over a longer period of time, from a minimum of one month to four months, with daily sessions of 10 minutes each. If there is no noticeable improvement of the condition, you should seek the advice of your doctor.

The amount of downward pressure that you apply depends on whether you want to treat or diagnose a condition. If you are treating a known condition, apply light-to-medium pressure on the palm. If you want to diagnose a condition, you will need to apply medium-to-strong pressure on the palm. As a tool, you can use a small wooden stick with a flattened head (similar to the tip of the thumb).

The diagram below shows energy-draining treatment.

Figure 8

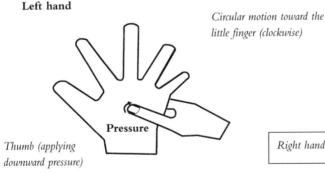

Left hand

Circular motion toward the little finger (clockwise)

Pressure

Thumb (applying downward pressure)

Right hand: Counterclockwise motion

The 10-Step Program

The 10-step program works with all the reflex zones of the hand and therefore treats all organs and body parts. It can also be used for diagnostic purposes.

For a complete treatment using the 10-step program, you need to allocate 25 to 40 minutes. The list below shows the respective organs and body parts in the left column and the corresponding reflex zones of the hand in the right column.

If you experience pain during the treatment, a disorder is present and you should continue to massage the respective zone one to five minutes longer.

1. Spinal column	Zone 1/A, B, C
2. Head, face, neck, shoulder and arm	Zones 1, 2, 3, 4, 5/A, B
3. Heart, heart-related zone, lungs	Zones 1, 2, 3, 4, 5/B
4. Stomach, pancreas, spleen, gallbladder, liver, large intestine, small intestine	Zones 1, 2, 3, 4, 5/B, C
5. Kidneys, ureter, bladder	Zones 3, 2, 1/B, C
6. Pelvic region (sciatic nerve)	Zones 2, 3, 4, 5/C
7. Women: Ovaries, fallopian tubes, uterus	Zones 5, 4, 3, 2, 1/C
Men: Testicles, seminal duct, prostate gland	Zones 5, 4, 3, 2, 1/C
8. Hip joint, thigh, knee	Zones 3, 4/C
9. Muscular and lymphatic vessels	Zones 1, 2, 3, 4, 5/A, B, C
10. Solar plexus (for a calming effect)	Zones 2, 3/B

The Lines of the Hand as Helpful Landmarks

With the help of the lines of the hand, the different reflex zones can be found quite easily, facilitating treatment (see Figures 9 and 10).

First, there are the lines along the finger joints. These indicate the reflex zones of the head and face. Between the metacarpophalangeal finger joints, the so-called webs can be found. The space between the thumb and the index finger is taken up mainly by the reflex zone of the heart, whereas the webs between the remaining fingers contain the reflex zones of the upper lymph ducts.

The character line of the left hand is the guideline for the heart-related zone, whereas the character line of the right hand forms the guideline for the lungs. The heart line is a guideline for the kidneys, but also for the spleen on the left hand, and for the liver and gallbladder on the right hand.

One of the shortest lines is the base line of the thumb, which separates the head-and-neck area from the chest-and-upper-stomach area. Consequently, the stomach reflex zone is situated just beside this line. If you work your way through the digestive organs, you will cross the life line and reach the end of the heart line. There, you will find the pancreas and spleen on the left hand and the liver and gallbladder on the right hand. From this point onward, you will find the soft parts, such as the large and small intestines. The wrist line forms the lower border. Therefore, the rectum reflex zone can be found on the left hand above the wrist line on the side of the thumb.

The heart line and the life line approach each other as they run toward the index finger; below the index finger and the middle finger, there may be a joining of the two lines, or they may run parallel without ever touching. In this triangle between the heart and the life lines, the solar plexus can be found.

The organs that are located in the pelvic region can be found between the wrist line and the arm base line. On the thumb side, on both the left and the right hands, there is the bladder, and on the little finger side, on both hands, there is the reflex point for the sciatic nerve.

The back of the hand doesn't have lines like the palm does, but other "landmarks" can easily be located by touch (see Figure 11). These are the two bones of the arm that end at the wrist: the radius on the thumb side and the ulna on the little finger side. In this area, the reflex zones for all the lower abdominal organs can be found, as can those for the thighs as far as the knees. In women, the ovaries are located above the ulna and the uterus above the radius. They are connected by the fallopian tubes. In men, the testicles are situated above the ulna and the prostate gland above the radius. The link between the two is the seminal duct.

In addition, the hips, thighs, and knees are located in this area. The hips can be found next to the ovaries (testicles, with men), and the knees are situated at the wrist, just between the ulna and the radius. The reflex zone of the thighs forms the connection between the hips and the knees.

The remaining area on the back of the hand is taken up by the muscles and the lymph ducts of the entire body.

Lines of the Hand

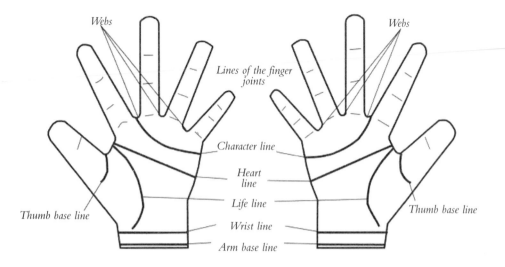

Webs

Webs

Lines of the finger joints

Character line

Heart line

Life line

Thumb base line

Thumb base line

Wrist line

Arm base line

Figure 9

Lines of the Hand and Their Directly Affiliated Reflex Zones

Left hand   **Right hand**

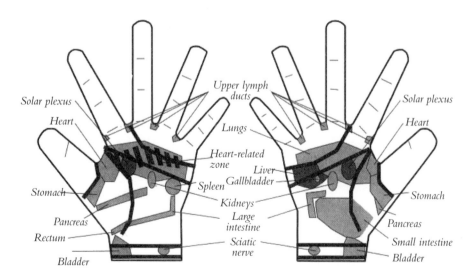

Solar plexus

Solar plexus

Heart

Heart

Upper lymph ducts

Lungs

Heart-related zone

Liver

Stomach

Spleen

Gallbladder

Stomach

Kidneys

Pancreas

Large intestine

Pancreas

Rectum

Small intestine

Bladder

Sciatic nerve

Bladder

Figure 10

Distinctive Reflex Zones on the Back of the Hand

Left hand   **Right hand**

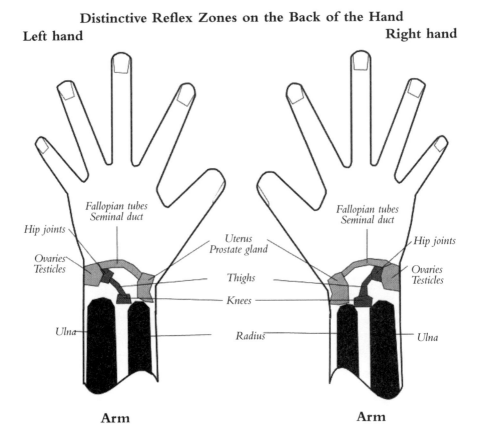

Figure 11

The Practice of Hand Reflexology: Clinical Pictures

On the following page, you will find an overview of the conditions that you can treat using hand reflexology. They are divided into subchapters according to which area of the body or which organ they affect, and, within these subchapters, they appear in alphabetical order. For each condition, the causes are explained, typical symptoms are listed, and the most important conventional therapies are given. In a box at the bottom of the page, reference is made to particular dangers or other important aspects.

If you only skimmed the previous chapter or didn't read it at all, we recommend that you do read it, and perhaps more than once, before you go on. Only when you are familiar with the basic theory underlying reflexology, and have mastered the massage technique, can you start with its practical applications. Here, you have two possibilities: You can use the reflex zones as a diagnostic aid to help you find the individual organs requiring attention, or, by massaging the reflex points, you can treat any condition that you may have discovered.

Although the reflex zones of the hand are valuable tools for determining which organ may be affected by a certain complaint, the diagnosis that you arrive at should not be regarded as final proof of the presence of certain conditions. If you suspect that a serious illness may be present, it's important to ask your doctor to verify your diagnosis.

For the massage of the hand reflex zones, you will find diagrams of hands for each condition showing the main reflex zones and the secondary zones. Treat the individual zones according to the table at the bottom of the page, using the technique specified—that is, either building up or draining energy. For quick reference, the direction of the massage, either on the palm or the back of the hand, is indicated by a turning arrow.

During the massage, the initial pain from applying pressure on the reflex zone should decrease if you are using the correct technique. Often an existing complaint will improve at the same rate. If there is no improvement, or if the condition is exacerbated, you should change your massage technique. If there is still no improvement, then check your diagnosis and reconsider whether or not this type of therapy is suitable.

1. Head-and-Neck Area

1.1 Catarrh of the upper respiratory tract
1.2 Ear complaints
1.3 Eye complaints
1.4 Headaches
1.5 Paranasal sinusitis
1.6 Swollen lymph nodes
1.7 Tonsillitis
1.8 Toothache

2. Chest Organs

2.1 Acute and chronic bronchitis
2.2 Arrhythmia
2.3 Bronchial asthma
2.4 Cardiac pain (angina pectoris)
2.5 Emphysema
2.6 Heart attack aftercare
2.7 Weakened heart

3. Abdominal Organs

3.1 Abdominal cramps
3.2 Bile duct disorders
3.3 Constipation
3.4 Diarrhea
3.5 Flatulence
3.6 Heartburn
3.7 Hemorrhoids
3.8 Liver disorders
3.9 Pancreas complaints
3.10 Stomach pain

4. Urinary and Sexual Organs

4.1 Bladder complaints
4.2 Disorders of the ovaries and fallopian tubes
4.3 Disorders of the uterus
4.4 Female infertility
4.5 Kidney disorders
4.6 Male impotence
4.7 Mammary gland disorders
4.8 Menopausal problems
4.9 Menstrual problems
4.10 Problems during pregnancy
4.11 Prostate complaints

5. Spinal Column and Limbs

5.1 Complaints of the lower spinal column
5.2 Complaints of the upper spinal column
5.3 Disorders of the knee joint
5.4 Hip complaints
5.5 Injury aftercare
5.6 Muscular disorders
5.7 Rheumatic disorders
5.8 Shoulder pain
5.9 Tennis elbow
5.10 Varicose veins

6. The Nervous System

6.1 Dizziness
6.2 Lack of concentration
6.3 Neurasthenia (nervousness)
6.4 Neuritis
6.5 Paralysis
6.6 Stroke

7. Skin

7.1 Eczema
7.2 Itching
7.3 Nettle rash
7.4 Neurodermatitis
7.5 Psoriasis

8. Complex Clinical Pictures

8.1 Allergies
8.2 Burnout syndrome
8.3 Circulatory disorders
8.4 Circulatory weakness
8.5 Depression
8.6 Diabetes
8.7 Excess weight
8.8 Giving up smoking
8.9 Hypertension
8.10 Migraines
8.11 Pain from scars
8.12 Sleep disorders
8.13 Weakened resistance to infection

1. Head-and-Neck Area

1.1 Catarrh of the upper respiratory tract

1.2 Ear complaints

1.3 Eye complaints

1.4 Headaches

1.5 Paranasal sinusitis

1.6 Swollen lymph nodes

1.7 Tonsillitis

1.8 Toothache

1.1 Catarrh of the upper respiratory tract

Definition

Catarrh (from the Greek *katarrheo*, meaning "flowing down") refers to an inflammation of the mucous membranes with an increased production of liquid secretion. All parts of the body with a mucous membrane can be affected. Commonly, the term "catarrh" refers to the upper respiratory tract, which comprises the following:
- Nasal cavity
- Nasal sinuses
- Mouth and throat
- Larynx
- Windpipe and bronchial tubes

It is usually caused by pathogens that attack locally and trigger an inflammation. However, strong physical or chemical stimuli can provoke a similar reaction.

Symptoms

In addition to feeling generally unwell, you may have these symptoms:
- Swelling of the mucous membranes
- Watery or purulent secretions
- Narrowing of the respiratory tract
- Fever, exhaustion, tiredness

Treatment Guidelines

Under normal circumstances, the body possesses all the equipment it needs to effectively fight pathogens. Before you start taking medicines, you should therefore undertake some general measures to support your body:
- Sufficient sleep, a sensible diet, no physical exertion

A treatment of the symptoms only comes second:
- Inhalation, heat treatment
- Localized disinfecting (gargling with a saline solution, cleaning of teeth)
- Boosting the immune system with herbal remedies such as echinacea or thuja
- Lowering fever:
  With cold compresses or washes
  With medications such as paracetamol, acetylsalicylic acid, or quinine
- Expectorant and anti-inflammatory remedies:
  Chemical: acetyl cysteine, ambroxol
  Plant-based: thyme, ivy, liquorice, peppermint, eucalyptus, coltsfoot

---

Important!
Treatment with antibiotics can only be prescribed by your doctor. Antibiotics show no effect against common viral infections, but with serious bacterial infections accompanied by a high fever (for example, with scarlet fever or rheumatic fever), antibiotics are extremely effective in preventing damage to important organs.

CATARRH OF THE UPPER RESPIRATORY TRACT

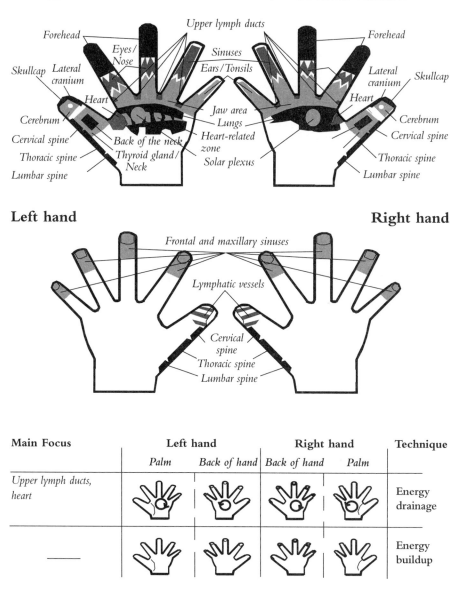

Upper lymph ducts

Forehead

Eyes/Nose

Sinuses

Ears/Tonsils

Skullcap Lateral cranium

Forehead

Lateral cranium Skullcap

Heart

Heart

Cerebrum

Jaw area

Lungs

Cerebrum

Cervical spine

Back of the neck

Heart-related zone

Cervical spine

Thoracic spine

Thyroid gland/Neck

Solar plexus

Thoracic spine

Lumbar spine

Lumbar spine

Left hand   **Right hand**

Frontal and maxillary sinuses

Lymphatic vessels

Cervical spine

Thoracic spine

Lumbar spine

Main Focus	Left hand		Right hand		Technique
	Palm	Back of hand	Back of hand	Palm	
Upper lymph ducts, heart					Energy drainage
————					Energy buildup

37

1.2 Ear complaints

Definition

The ear is divided up into three sections, anatomically and functionally:
- Outer ear: auricle, auditory canal, eardrum
- Middle ear: eardrum, tympanic cavity, auditory ossicles, tube
- Inner ear: cochlea (hearing organ), labyrinth (balance organ)

The outer ear is designed to absorb sound and transmit it on to the middle ear, where the eardrum begins to vibrate. These vibrations are then transmitted to the auditory ossicles and, after being amplified mechanically, conducted to the inner ear. The cochlea, the actual hearing sensor, is filled with a fluid that stimulates the hair cells of the hearing organ and creates a nerve signal.

Symptoms

Complaints of the outer ear usually involve inflammatory processes with:
- Pain, fever, secretion from the auditory canal

If the mucous membrane of the pharynx is swollen, the narrow tube becomes blocked and disables the equalization of pressure between the pharyngeal cavity and the middle ear. This leads to:
- Pain, outward bulging of the eardrum, impaired hearing
- Accumulation of fluid and mucus, as well as purulent bacteria

The inner ear is often affected by infections that spread from the middle ear. In addition, frequently there is disturbed circulation, a problem to which the nerve cells of the hearing organ are particularly susceptible. Damage to the inner ear is characterized by:
- Dizziness, impaired hearing with regard to particular pitches
- Complete loss of hearing (acute hearing loss), constant ear noise (tinnitus)

However, if one auditory canal is blocked by a plug, the imbalance of stimulation to the hearing organ may result in similar complaints.

Treatment Guidelines

The treatment depends on the cause of the condition. In the case of inflammatory processes of the outer and middle ear, general treatment of the infection (see 1.1 Catarrh) is supported by using anti-inflammatory remedies locally and, if necessary, administering painkillers. There is disagreement regarding localized treatment with antibiotics. Ear infections that are accompanied by a high fever and pain should be treated by a doctor. If complaints are only minor, it will often suffice to treat the symptoms through:
- Measures to reduce the swelling of the nasal-and-pharyngeal area, heat therapy

> **Important!**
> Acute loss of hearing or deafness by shock waves requires immediate and intensive treatment, because damaged auditory cells die rapidly and cannot be replaced. The result is a permanent loss of hearing.

EAR COMPLAINTS

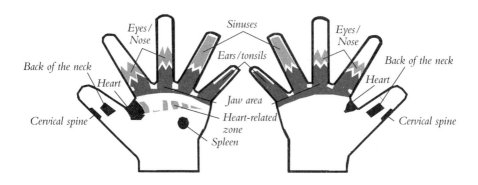

Left hand   **Right hand**

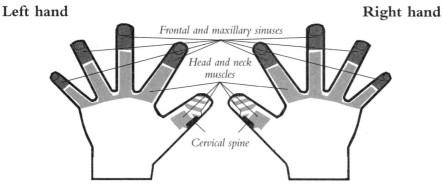

Main Focus	Left hand		Right hand		Technique
	Palm	*Back of hand*	*Back of hand*	*Palm*	
Ears/tonsils, jaw area					Energy drainage
——					Energy buildup

1.3 Eye complaints

Definition:

The term "eye complaints" does not refer to a particular condition. The eye as a sensory organ, with its tear ducts, optic nerve, and visual center, forms a functional unit in the brain. The causes of impaired vision can lie in any of the areas in this unit.

The eye itself consists of mechanical optical components at the front, including the cornea, the iris, and the pupil. At the back of the eye, light hits the retina's highly sensitive sensors. From there, the optic nerve extends to the cranial base and into the central area of the brain, where the signals are further transmitted to the visual cortex, producing an image.

Impaired vision can be caused by an illness of the eye itself, but also by a disturbance in the processing and the perception of visual stimuli in the brain. The sensors in the retina are brain cells and have only a limited ability to regenerate once they have been damaged. Impaired vision should therefore always be examined by an ophthalmologist. If the retina has been severely damaged, scars will form during the healing process, resulting in a loss of eyesight. Injuries to the front of the eye also need to be treated immediately and by a qualified practitioner. Inflammation of the cornea due to pathogens or foreign bodies could lead to clouding and thus permanently impaired vision.

Symptoms

Important symptoms of eye complaints:
- Impaired vision
- Headaches
- Feeling of pressure within the eye, burning sensation
- Secretion of tears

Treatment Guidelines

Before you attempt self-treatment, you should be examined by a doctor in order to rule out any serious eye conditions. Minor complaints can be treated as follows, depending on the symptoms:
- Cold compresses or washing of the eye
- Eye drops to reduce irritation
- Relaxation techniques
- Avoidance of unnecessary light stimuli, such as strobe lights in discotheques or the glare from TV

> **Important!**
> Conditions of the retina require immediate examination and treatment by an ophthalmologist. TV sets and computer screens emit strong visual stimuli; regular breaks and relaxation periods can help to avoid problems. Diabetes can cause premature damage of the retina; this is one of the reasons why it's important for diabetics to undergo regular checkups.

EYE COMPLAINTS

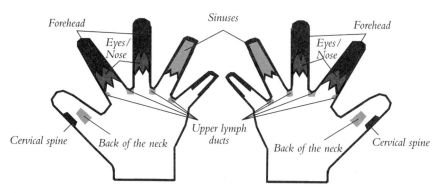

Forehead   Sinuses   Forehead

Eyes/Nose   Eyes/Nose

Cervical spine   Back of the neck   Upper lymph ducts   Back of the neck   Cervical spine

Left hand   **Right hand**

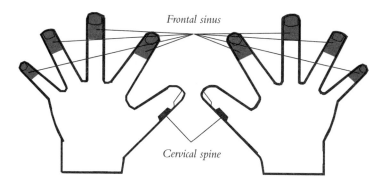

Frontal sinus

Cervical spine

Main Focus	Left hand		Right hand		Technique
	Palm	Back of hand	Back of hand	Palm	
Frontal sinus, increased intraocular pressure					Energy drainage
Other eye and nose complaints					Energy buildup

41

1.4 Headaches

Definition

Headaches can have a number of causes. Most commonly, sufferers experience dull waves of pain accompanied by a sensation of pressure in the head. Migraines are a particular type of headache characterized by severe, stabbing pains, often on one side only and accompanied by nausea and circulatory problems. Tugging pains that radiate from the cervical spine into the back of the neck are very common too. They are caused by a mechanical irritation of the nerve roots where they emerge from the spine. The sensory organs—for example, the eyes, the ears, and the oral cavity, especially the teeth—may also be at the source of headaches. In addition, localized and general inflammatory reactions, such as sinusitis or a high fever, may be accompanied by headaches. Meningitis and inflammation of the brain itself are much rarer, but extremely serious. An increased pressure inside the skull—for example, due to bleeding—may cause headaches as well.

Symptoms

Headaches are very common and don't always require a diagnosis and special therapy. However, if you experience any of the points below, without an apparent cause, you should always consult your doctor:

- Sudden, persistent headaches that are significantly stronger than any headaches experienced previously
- Persistent headache after extreme physical exertion
- One-sided pain occurring for the first time
- Headache accompanied by a stiff neck and a fever
- Headache accompanied by dysesthesia (impairment of sensitivity, especially to touch), paralysis, or reduced consciousness

Treatment Guidelines

A light headache often doesn't require special treatment. The following measures may relieve the symptoms:

- Cold compresses, taking it easy, avoiding light and sound irritation

In chronic cases, these measures may be useful:

- Relaxation techniques, stress management, exercise

Painkillers should just be used rarely and in a controlled manner:

- General: paracetamol, acetylsalicylic acid, codeine (often in conjunction with other active ingredients)
- For migraines: ergotamine preparations
- For muscular tension: chloromezanone, tetrazepam, baclofen

Important!
The continuous use of painkillers can quickly lead to at least a psychogenic dependency. Today, we have become increasingly sensitive to pain. Yet pain is important for a healthy, normal physical awareness and should not be suppressed automatically.

HEADACHES

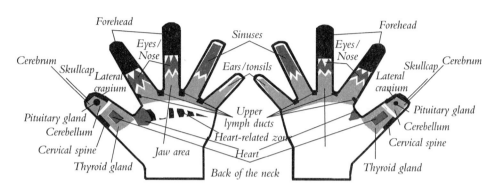

Forehead · Sinuses · Forehead
Eyes/Nose · Eyes/Nose
Cerebrum · Skullcap · Lateral cranium · Ears/tonsils · Skullcap · Cerebrum
Lateral cranium
Pituitary gland · Upper lymph ducts · Pituitary gland
Cerebellum · Heart-related zone · Cerebellum
Cervical spine · Cervical spine
Jaw area · Heart
Thyroid gland · Thyroid gland
Back of the neck

Left hand   **Right hand**

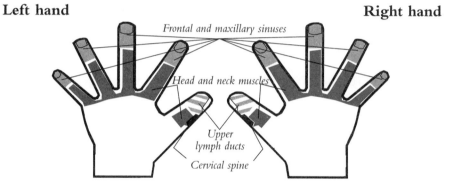

Frontal and maxillary sinuses

Head and neck muscles

Upper lymph ducts

Cervical spine

Main Focus	Left hand		Right hand		Technique
	Palm	*Back of hand*	*Back of hand*	*Palm*	
Heart, neck muscles					Energy drainage
———					Energy buildup

43

1.5 Paranasal sinusitis

Definition

The facial bones that make up the forehead and the upper jaw possess cavities that are connected with the nasal passage, from where they are ventilated. The walls of these paranasal sinuses are lined with mucous membranes that secrete mucus into the nasal passage. If these membranes are swollen, the entrance to the sinuses may be blocked, hindering mucus secretion and ventilation. The roots of the molars reach into the maxillary sinus; therefore, an inflammation of the teeth can affect the sinus. Likewise, if the maxillary sinus is inflamed, the roots of the molars can be affected, leading to toothache. If paranasal sinusitis occurs frequently, this can be caused by:

- Infection due to pathogens
- Reduced ventilation as a result of impaired nasal breathing
- Scar formation from chronic inflammation

Symptoms

Depending on the cause and the severity of the inflammation, it is possible to have these symptoms:

- Pressure and pain above and below the eyes
- Swollen nasal lining, secretion
- Fever, exhaustion
- Toothache

Treatment Guidelines

Minor cases of sinusitis are treated according to their symptoms. Physical therapy and essential oils bring quick relief:

- Infrared light
- Inhalation—for example, with peppermint, eucalyptus, or chamomile

Treatment of the mucous membranes:

- Chemical: ambroxol, acetyl cysteine
- Plant-based: myrrh, citrus oils

If the inflammation is accompanied by a high fever and suppuration, your doctor will undoubtedly prescribe antibiotics. It is important to complete the full course of treatment, unless you have a bad reaction to the antibiotics.

Important!
Persistent and severe suppuration of the paranasal sinuses can result in serious problems affecting the teeth, the eyes, the soft parts of the face, and the intracranial area, including the brain and the meninges (the membranes enveloping the brain). If the condition is accompanied by a fever and suppuration, and does not improve within seven to 10 days, you must seek medical advice.

PARANASAL SINUSITUS

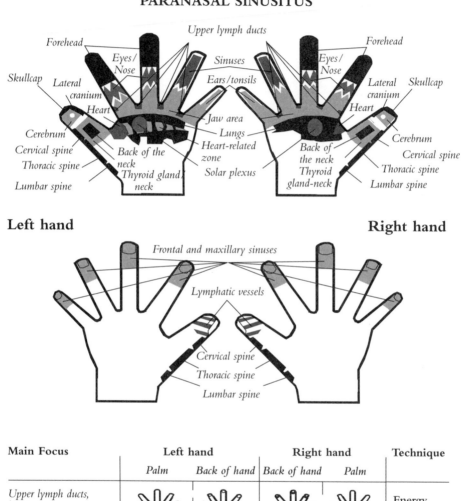

Forehead — Eyes/Nose — Upper lymph ducts — Sinuses — Forehead — Eyes/Nose

Skullcap — Lateral cranium — Heart — Ears/tonsils — Lateral cranium — Skullcap — Heart

Cerebrum — Cervical spine — Thoracic spine — Lumbar spine — Back of the neck — Jaw area — Lungs — Heart-related zone — Solar plexus — Thyroid gland, neck — Back of the neck — Thyroid gland-neck — Cerebrum — Cervical spine — Thoracic spine — Lumbar spine

Left hand   **Right hand**

Frontal and maxillary sinuses

Lymphatic vessels

Cervical spine
Thoracic spine
Lumbar spine

Main Focus	Left hand		Right hand		Technique
	Palm	Back of hand	Back of hand	Palm	
Upper lymph ducts, heart, sinuses					Energy drainage
————					Energy buildup

1.6 Swollen lymph nodes

Definition

Swollen lymph nodes (lymphadenitis) indicate a reaction by the immune system. When an inflammatory reaction is due to pathogens, for instance, they stimulate the white blood cells that travel along the lymph ducts to the lymph nodes, where they activate the body's defenses further. This reaction is characterized by an inflammatory swelling of the lymph nodes. Some lymphatic cells are capable of absorbing foreign substances and pathogens and transporting them to the lymphatic organs to be destroyed. The local lymph nodes are the place where the lymph ducts of a particular region of the body come together. They drain by way of several different lymph nodes and enter the bloodstream at the vena cava. The liver and the spleen are also major lymphatic organs connected to the bloodstream.

Symptoms

The swelling of lymph nodes is a nonspecific reaction initially and does not allow for any conclusions as to its causes. The individual lymph nodes, however, indicate which region of the body is affected. This becomes particularly obvious with the arms and the legs, where the auxiliary and inguinal glands are located.

The swelling of lymph nodes is a frequent and necessary reaction, and usually dies down within two to three weeks. If the swelling remains beyond this time, the causes should be investigated. Painful swelling of lymph nodes, in particular, should be examined by a doctor immediately.

Treatment Guidelines

Normally, swollen lymph nodes don't require any specific treatment if the cause has been established and, if necessary, treated. However, these measures can be helpful:
- Warm compresses or packs (only during the initial stages)
- Cool compresses or packs (in the case of severe and chronic swelling)
- Anti-inflammatory medications:
  Chemical: diclofenac, ibuprofen, piroxicam
  Biological: heparin
  Plant-based: horse chestnut, witch hazel, arnica, chamomile

---

Important!
Chronic, often painful swelling of the lymph nodes is characteristic of diseases of the white blood cells (leukemia), tuberculosis, tumors, and other deficiencies of the immune system (for example, AIDS).

SWOLLEN LYMPH NODES

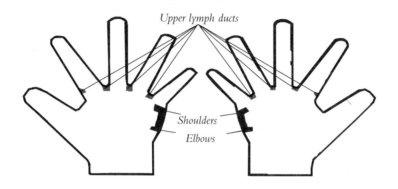

Upper lymph ducts

Shoulders
Elbows

Left hand   **Right hand**

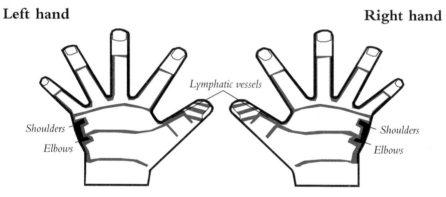

Lymphatic vessels

Shoulders   Shoulders
Elbows   Elbows

Main Focus	Left hand		Right hand		Technique
	Palm	*Back of hand*	*Back of hand*	*Palm*	
All lymphatic vessels					Energy drainage
——					Energy buildup

1.7 Tonsillitis

Definition

The tonsils (from the Latin *tonsillae*) are made up of lymphatic tissue and are found in the area of the nose, mouth, and throat. They are similar to the lymph nodes in other areas of the body. There are different types of tonsils: The larger ones are the palatine and pharyngeal tonsils, the smaller and less significant ones the laryngeal and lingual tonsils.

As with the lymph nodes, an inflammatory swelling of the lymphatic tissue of the tonsils is a normal and necessary reaction against intruding pathogens. A persisting inflammatory state over a period of time, however, will result in growths and scarring of the tissue. If the inflammation is severe, purulent disintegration can occur. Where there is scar tissue or purulent cavities, bacteria can no longer be fought effectively and can cause infections to flare up again and again. Streptococci and staphylococci are the most dangerous, because they can cause serious inflammation of the heart valves, cardiac muscle, kidneys, and joints.

- Adenoids: growths off the pharyngeal tonsils, causing displacement of the rear nasal passage (impaired nasal breathing)
- Angina tonsillaris (tonsillitis): inflammation of the palatine tonsils, causing them to swell and thereby narrow the back of the mouth (difficulty when swallowing)

Symptoms

An inflammation of the tonsils (tonsillitis) due to pathogens can lead to:
- Fever, generally feeling unwell
- Difficulty when swallowing, pain
- Swollen lymph nodes and soft parts in the neck
- Impaired breathing

Treatment Guidelines

If the inflammation and the enlargement of the tonsils are minor and not accompanied by a fever and suppuration, there are a number of ways of treating the symptoms:
- Cool compresses around the neck, creams for lymphatic drainage
- Localized disinfecting (saline solutions) and oral hygiene
- Astringents (sage, chamomile, hexetidin)
- Boosting the immune system (echinacea, thuja)

If tonsillitis is accompanied by a high temperature and suppuration, it is necessary to consult your doctor, who should prescribe a course of antibiotics.

Important!
In small children, growths and suppuration of the tonsils can quickly lead to a constriction of the already narrow pharyngeal area and may make breathing difficult. Tonsillitis in children should therefore be treated early.

TONSILLITIS

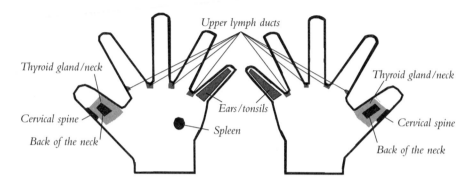

Left hand   **Right hand**

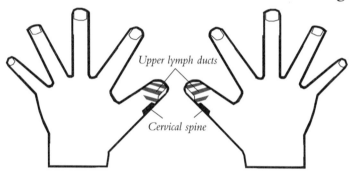

Main Focus	Left hand		Right hand		Technique
	Palm	Back of hand	Back of hand	Palm	
Ears/tonsils, upper lymph ducts					Energy drainage
———					Energy buildup

1.8 Toothache

Definition

Toothache is frequently caused by conditions affecting the teeth, such as:
- Cavities
- Periodontosis
- Inflammation of the tooth root

Yet toothache can also be induced by illnesses affecting adjoining areas, such as:
- Paranasal sinusitis
- Inflammation of the trigeminal nerve

Owing to the close proximity to the brain, toothache is always experienced as very intense, causing people to seek fast and effective therapies.

Symptoms

There are different kinds of toothache, enabling us to draw conclusions as to their causes:
- Sensitivity to hot and cold stimuli is characteristic of exposed necks of teeth—for instance, in the case of periodontosis or damaged tooth enamel.
- Sensitivity to sweet foods indicates decay of tooth enamel as the result of cavities.
- If pain radiates into the entire jaw or half the face, neuralgia may be present.
- Loss of strength and pain when chewing can be caused by a condition affecting the jaw joint.

Treatment Guidelines

With toothache, treatment of the causes is paramount, so you should visit your dentist as soon as possible. Painkillers will dampen the pain, but they won't remove its cause. Because toothache usually means quite severe pain, it is advisable to use a medication that contains painkillers and anti-inflammatory agents, such as the following:
- Paracetamol, acetylsalicylic acid, codeine, diclofenac, naproxen, ibuprofen

---

Important!
Cleaning your teeth regularly and properly and choosing the right kinds of food will help prevent tooth decay and related complaints.

TOOTHACHE

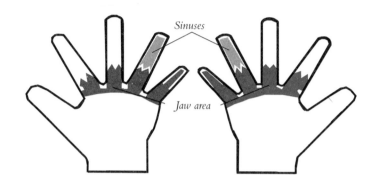

Sinuses

Jaw area

Left hand

Right hand

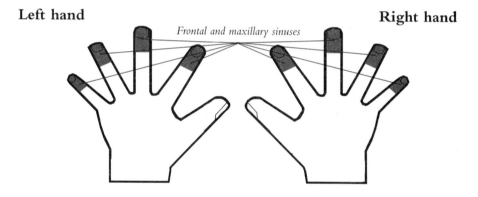

Frontal and maxillary sinuses

Main Focus	Left hand		Right hand		Technique
	Palm	*Back of hand*	*Back of hand*	*Palm*	
Jaw area					Energy drainage
——					Energy buildup

2. Chest Organs

2.1 Acute and chronic bronchitis

2.2 Arrhythmia

2.3 Bronchial asthma

2.4 Cardiac pain (angina pectoris)

2.5 Emphysema

2.6 Heart attack aftercare

2.7 Weakened heart

2.1 Acute and chronic bronchitis

Definition

Bronchitis (from the Greek *bronchos,* meaning "branches," and *itis,* meaning "inflammation") is an inflammatory illness of the respiratory system. Behind the sternum, the windpipe forks toward the two lungs and forms the main bronchi. These branch off into the lungs in the shape of trees. At the end of the smallest bronchial tubes are the alveoli, where the gas exchange takes place. The larger bronchial tubes are reinforced with cartilage braces, to prevent them from collapsing under the constant change of pressure from breathing. The walls of the smaller bronchial tubes are equipped with muscle fibers that allow them to adjust their width. This controls the distribution of the air in the lungs. On the inside, the bronchial tubes are furnished with cilia and protected by mucus.

The following are the most frequent causes of bronchitis:
- Irritants such as chemicals or smoke
- Pathogens like bacteria, viruses, or fungi
- Physical irritation such as cold or humidity

Symptoms

Acute bronchitis is characterized by:
- Increased mucus production, expectoration
- Greenish-yellow mucus
- An urge to cough
- Burning pain in the chest after coughing
- General symptoms of infection, fever

Bronchitis is considered chronic if the symptoms persist over a long period of time or become permanent. Chronic inflammation leads to:
- Convulsive narrowing of the small bronchial tubes (see 2.3, Bronchial asthma)
- Overly inflated lungs (see 2.5, Emphysema)
- More difficult breathing, due to greater resistance in the respiratory tract, a reduced area for gas exchange, and a loss of elasticity

Treatment Guidelines

Pathogens should be attacked with:
- Antibiotics
- Expectorants (ambroxol, acetyl cysteine, ivy, thyme)
- Immune stimulants (echinacea, thuja, bacteria vaccine)

In addition, it's important to ensure that the inflammation dies down completely. The inflammatory process often doesn't cause any complaints, but in the long term it can lead to premature aging of the lungs (see 2.5, Emphysema).

> **Important!**
> With bronchitis, the coughed-up mucus sometimes contains blood. This symptom always needs to be taken seriously, and you should consult your doctor every time to determine the cause.

ACUTE AND CHRONIC BRONCHITIS

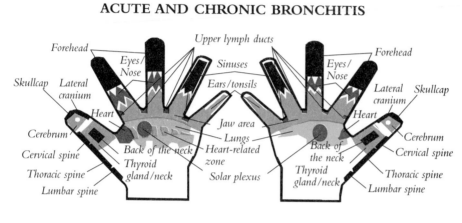

Forehead
Eyes/Nose
Skullcap
Lateral cranium
Heart
Cerebrum
Cervical spine
Thoracic spine
Lumbar spine

Upper lymph ducts
Sinuses
Ears/tonsils
Jaw area
Lungs
Back of the neck
Heart-related zone
Thyroid gland/neck
Solar plexus

Forehead
Eyes/Nose
Lateral cranium
Skullcap
Heart
Cerebrum
Cervical spine
Thoracic spine
Lumbar spine
Back of the neck
Thyroid gland/neck

Left hand   **Right hand**

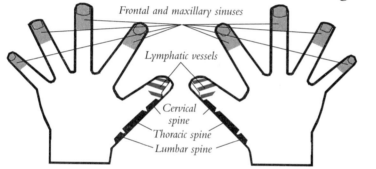

Frontal and maxillary sinuses

Lymphatic vessels

Cervical spine
Thoracic spine
Lumbar spine

Main Focus	Left hand		Right hand		Technique
	Palm	*Back of hand*	*Back of hand*	*Palm*	
Upper lymph ducts, heart, lungs					Energy drainage
————					Energy buildup

55

2.2 Arrhythmia

Definition

The heart has a network similar to that of the nervous system, and it produces independent electrical impulses, which it then transmits to the individual parts of the heart. The pulse rate can be influenced from the outside via the nerves (for example, the vagus nerve) and by hormones (such as adrenaline). Arrhythmia can be brought on by external triggers, or the cause can be found in the heart itself. Possible external causes include the following:
- Hormonal imbalance of the thyroid gland
- Mineral imbalances
- Stress

In the heart itself, arrhythmia can be caused by:
- Inflammation
- Lack of oxygen
- Scars
- High blood pressure

Symptoms

Arrhythmia can affect the pace or the regularity of the heartbeat:
- Heartbeat is even and too fast (tachycardia)
- Heartbeat is even and too slow (bradycardia)
- Heartbeat stops for a period of time (asystolia)
- Individual, irregular additional heartbeats (extrasystole)
- Persistently irregular heartbeat (arrhythmia)

Arrhythmia rarely causes serious complaints. Occasionally, there can be these symptoms:
- Palpitations
- Extrasystole
- Inner unrest
- Signs of a weak heart

Treatment Guidelines

The treatment of arrhythmia depends on the cause. Most cases of arrhythmia are not life-threatening and just occur temporarily. Only a doctor can establish with certainty if and what treatment is necessary. Always consider the following possible causes of the complaint:
- Medications that you may currently be taking
- Thyroid problems, goiter
- Mental state

Important!
If you suffer from an infection and experience arrhythmia, this may indicate an inflammation of the cardiac muscle. In the case of known coronary heart disease, arrhythmia may be caused by a heart attack.

ARRHYTHMIA

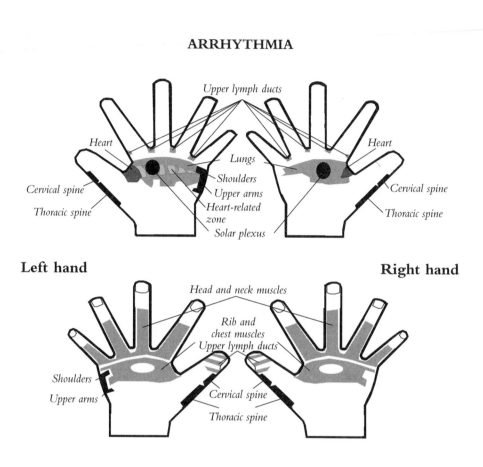

Upper lymph ducts

Heart

Lungs

Shoulders
Upper arms
Heart-related zone
Solar plexus

Cervical spine

Thoracic spine

Heart

Cervical spine

Thoracic spine

Left hand

Right hand

Head and neck muscles

Rib and chest muscles

Upper lymph ducts

Shoulders

Upper arms

Cervical spine

Thoracic spine

Main Focus	Left hand		Right hand		Technique
	Palm	Back of hand	Back of hand	Palm	
Heart-related zone					Energy drainage
Heart					Energy buildup

2.3 Bronchial asthma

Definition

Bronchial asthma (from the Greek *asthma,* meaning "narrowing") is a condition of the respiratory system. The main symptom of this condition is difficulty in breathing, which is due to a narrowing of the bronchial tubes that results in greater resistance when exhaling. The lungs become overly inflated, and the exchangeable amount of gases is reduced. As a result, breathing activity increases. In severe cases, the blood is not supplied with enough oxygen and carbon dioxide is not exhaled sufficiently, despite the increased rate in breathing. A lack of oxygen and excess blood acidity can trigger serious disturbances in the body.

The causes for convulsion of the bronchial tubes can be internal or external:
- Internal: usually chronic inflammation of the bronchial tubes with a heightened disposition toward convulsions or an increased formation of phlegm
- External: can be irritants or allergens (see 8.1, Allergies)

Symptoms

The symptoms of asthma can be present permanently or may occur intermittently. Severe attacks may become life-threatening for the sufferer within a relatively short period of time. These are some of the typical symptoms:
- Respiratory distress (dyspnea), accelerated breathing (tachypnea)
- Wheezing sound during breathing
- Pallor, blue tint to the lips (cyanosis)
- Accelerated pulse (tachycardia)
- Anxiety, restlessness

Treatment Guidelines

The treatment aims to reduce resistance in the respiratory tract, improve gas exchange, and stabilize circulation. However, an asthma attack that is just beginning can often be stopped with very simple measures:
- Special breathing techniques
- Relaxation techniques, aiming to deactivate the stress system

For acute attacks, people are given medications that dilate the bronchial tubes and are particularly effective when inhaled directly into the bronchial system. Among these medications are the following:
- Fenoterol, salbutamol, terbutaline, theophylline

If the inflammation of the bronchial tubes has become chronic, rigorous treatment with anti-inflammatory drugs, such as the inhalation of corticosteroids, is the only option to avoid serious aftereffects.

Important!
Relaxation techniques, breathing exercises, and alternative therapies such as reflexology cannot replace the necessary treatment of the root causes. Today, there are special examination methods that will show exactly what kind of treatment is useful and necessary.

BRONCHIAL ASTHMA

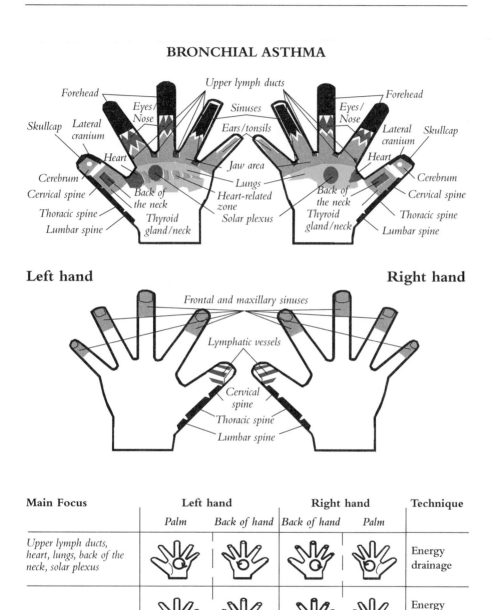

Main Focus	Left hand		Right hand		Technique
	Palm	Back of hand	Back of hand	Palm	
Upper lymph ducts, heart, lungs, back of the neck, solar plexus					Energy drainage
——					Energy buildup

2.4 Cardiac pain (angina pectoris)

Definition

Angina pectoris (from the Latin *angina,* meaning "narrowing," and *pectus,* meaning "chest") is a condition related to the heart and the circulatory system. It is characterized by pain in the chest caused by the cardiac muscle not receiving sufficient blood. This in turn is brought on by a narrowing of the coronary blood vessels—that is, coronary heart disease—or by convulsions of the coronary blood vessels as a result of external stimuli such as cold. If you rest adequately following an attack, the chances of a complete recovery and reduced pain are generally excellent. However, if the cardiac muscle still doesn't receive sufficient blood, its sensitive tissue will die because of a lack of oxygen and an accumulation of metabolic waste. This irreversible condition is called a heart attack.

Symptoms

- Stabbing, cramplike pain in the left side of the chest
- Pain often radiating into the left arm, the neck, the jaw, or the upper stomach
- Reduced physical stamina
- Vegetative signs such as pallor, cold sweats, restlessness
- Feelings of fear, often a fear of death

Treatment Guidelines

If the condition has been identified, the most important measure is taking emergency medicines right away:

- Nitrospray or nitro capsules

If the condition is occurring for the first time, a doctor should be consulted immediately. Meanwhile, it is helpful to:

- Take it easy
- Avoid excitement

Even if the symptoms disappear after a few minutes, you should still see your doctor without delay. There are a number of tests, such as an electrocardiogram or a blood count, that can determine the cause of the pain. If the pain persists for a while, you will need to be hospitalized.

Important!
The use of reflexology can never replace emergency medicines, nor can it deliver a reliable diagnosis. Reflexology should be used just with minor cases where the diagnosis is clear, and it should only support emergency medicines.

CARDIAC PAIN (ANGINA PECTORIS)

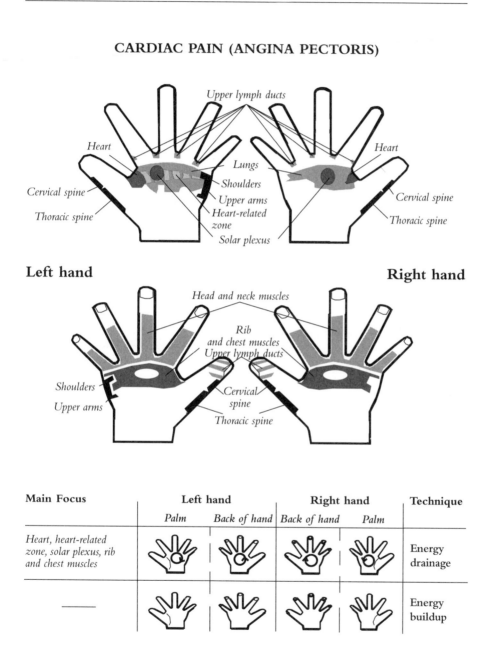

Left hand   **Right hand**

Main Focus	Left hand		Right hand		Technique
	Palm	*Back of hand*	*Back of hand*	*Palm*	
Heart, heart-related zone, solar plexus, rib and chest muscles					Energy drainage
———					Energy buildup

2.5 Emphysema

Definition

Emphysema ("inflation" in Greek) occurs after the lung tissue has been permanently damaged and has lost its elasticity due to excessive inflation or scarring. It is most commonly caused by chronic inflammation or diseases characterized by increased resistance in the respiratory tract such as asthma. The extent to which the lungs can inflate and deflate has a direct relationship with the amount of gases that can be exchanged. Elastic fibers in the lung tissue are responsible for the great elasticity of the lungs. Another important factor is the ability of the chest area to expand.

These are some of the common causes of pulmonary emphysema:
- Chronic bronchitis, such as in smokers
- Bronchial asthma
- Inhalation of dust particles
- Cystic fibrosis (a congenital disease with the production of viscous mucus)

Symptoms

Because gas exchange becomes more difficult, breathing is accelerated, especially during physical exertion, so that sufficient amounts of oxygen can be absorbed. If the reserves of the respiratory organs are depleted, there can be an occurrence of the following:
- Respiratory distress (dyspnea), depending on the level of exertion or strain
- Lack of oxygen in the blood, pallor
- Blood becoming enriched with carbon dioxide, lips developing a blue tint (cyanosis)
- Strain on circulation, accelerated pulse (tachycardia)
- Mucus in the lower sections of the lungs, an urge to cough, expectoration

Treatment Guidelines

Once the lungs have changed as a result of emphysema, treatment can alleviate the symptoms but no longer heal the disease. Still, you can't go wrong with the measures below:
- Avoiding all harmful factors such as smoke, dust, chemicals
- Treating infections early
- Treating inflammation rigorously and consistently—for example, by inhaling corticosteroids
- Learning special breathing techniques, and using them regularly
- Having regular checkups, even when you are free of symptoms

> **Important!**
> Emphysema often develops very slowly and is not marked by any pain. With smokers, a chronic cough with expectoration is never harmless, but signals a chronic inflammatory process in the respiratory tract. Once reduced performance of the respiratory organs becomes noticeable, the changes in the lung tissue are already far advanced.

EMPHYSEMA

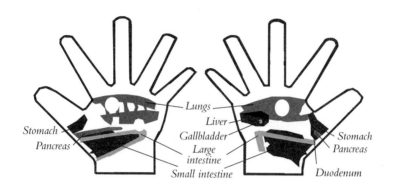

Stomach
Pancreas

Lungs
Liver
Gallbladder
Large intestine
Small intestine

Stomach
Pancreas

Duodenum

Left hand

Right hand

Main Focus	Left hand		Right hand		Technique
	Palm	*Back of hand*	*Back of hand*	*Palm*	
Lungs					Energy drainage
___					Energy buildup

2.6 Heart attack aftercare

Definition

A heart attack always results in the tissue of the cardiac muscle dying and causes permanent damage to the heart. A heart attack is caused by a lack of oxygen in the cardiac muscle tissue, usually because of a narrowed or blocked coronary vessel. Excessive strain on the cardiac muscle or severe inflammation can also lead to the dying of tissue. As a rule, a heart attack can be identified by stabbing, cramp-like pains that radiate into the left arm, the stomach, or the jaw (angina pectoris). During the acute phase, circulatory problems, arrhythmia, and a sense of being unwell are very common. The main cause for concern is that the patient may go into shock and suffer circulatory and organ failure. A heart attack may also go unnoticed, without obvious symptoms, only to be detected at a later date.

Heart attack patients always need to be hospitalized immediately. Modern technology can detect a blockage of the coronary vessels early by means of a catheter examination, and the condition can often be treated without surgery. The main aim is to limit the loss of cardiac muscle tissue. The earlier treatment begins, the better the chances of the patient's survival. With an acute attack, the problems persist.

Symptoms

The time after an acute attack is often characterized by:
■ Reduced physical stamina
■ Getting over the fear experienced during the acute attack
■ Reduced confidence in one's own body
■ Risk of complications such as another attack or arrhythmia
■ Carditis (inflammation of the heart muscle), enlargement of the heart, weakened heart

Treatment Guidelines

After an acute attack, patients begin rehabilitation. Important goals during this phase are the following:
◆ Stabilizing and exercising the circulatory system
◆ Reducing risk factors (excess weight, high blood pressure, smoking, diabetes, lack of exercise, disturbed fat metabolism)
◆ Restoring faith in one's own body
◆ Coping with depression

Important!
Depending on the type, the extent, and the course of the heart attack, different medications will be prescribed for aftercare. The treatment will be successful only if it is adhered to strictly. Alternative therapies can support conventional medical treatment, but they cannot replace it. Patients should never undertake changes to the treatment themselves—this should always be left to the doctor in charge.

HEART ATTACK AFTERCARE

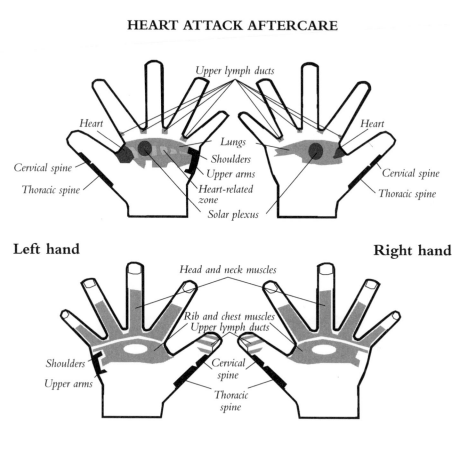

Main Focus	Left hand		Right hand		Technique
	Palm	Back of hand	Back of hand	Palm	
Heart-related zone, solar plexus	🖐	🖐	🖐	🖐	Energy drainage
	🖐	🖐	🖐	🖐	Energy buildup

2.7 Weakened heart

Definition

In medical terminology, a reduced performance of the heart is generally referred to as "cardiac insufficiency." It is usually caused by a problem in the heart itself:

- Valvular defect
- Myocardial insufficiency (inflammation, heart attack)
- Pericardial effusion
- Arrhythmia

If circulatory demands exceed the capabilities of the heart, even a healthy heart may show signs of weakness. Specific causes of weakness include the following:

- Severe loss of blood, shock after an accident, dehydration
- Kidney dysfunction
- High temperature
- Respiratory problems (for example, an asthma attack)

Symptoms

Impaired heart activity can affect the circulation of the body, including the lungs. These are the typical signs:

- Breathlessness, especially from exertion
- Fluid retention in tissue (edema), particularly around the ankles, around the eyelids, and in the lungs
- Accelerated heart rate
- Pallor, perspiration
- Urge to urinate, especially at night (nycturia)

Treatment Guidelines

In order to determine the causes, it's necessary to undertake low-impact examinations such as an ECG, an X ray of the chest, or an ultrasound of the heart. If the cause cannot be found in the heart itself, the causative illness has to be treated. Nevertheless, these measures will always be beneficial:

- Stamina training
- Reduction of risk factors (excess weight, smoking, alcohol, dietary fats)
- Normalization of blood pressure

The following medications can support heart activity:

- Chemical: diuretics such as furosemide, triamterene/hydrochlorothiazide; strengthening glycosides such as digoxin and digitoxin; preparations that affect the circulation such as ACE inhibitors, beta-blockers, calcium channel blockers
- Plant-based: hawthorn *(Crataegus oxyacantha)*, foxglove *(Digitalis purpurea)*, lily of the valley *(Convallaria majalis)*

Important!
The treatment of heart conditions is first and foremost the job of a doctor, as self-therapy is extremely risky. Alternative therapies can be used to support conventional treatment, depending on the causes.

WEAKENED HEART

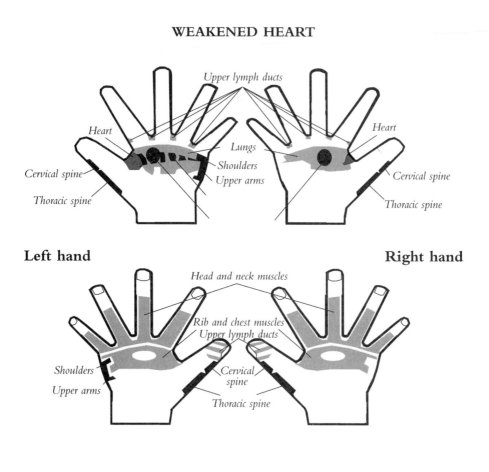

Upper lymph ducts

Heart

Lungs

Shoulders

Upper arms

Heart

Cervical spine

Thoracic spine

Cervical spine

Thoracic spine

Left hand

Right hand

Head and neck muscles

Rib and chest muscles

Upper lymph ducts

Shoulders

Cervical spine

Upper arms

Thoracic spine

Main Focus	Left hand		Right hand		Technique
	Palm	Back of hand	Back of hand	Palm	
Heart					Energy drainage
———					Energy buildup

3. Abdominal Organs

3.1 Abdominal cramps

3.2 Bile duct disorders

3.3 Constipation

3.4 Diarrhea

3.5 Flatulence

3.6 Heartburn

3.7 Hemorrhoids

3.8 Liver disorders

3.9 Pancreas complaints

3.10 Stomach pain

3.1 Abdominal cramps

Definition

Cramplike pains in the abdominal area signal an irritation of the highly sensitive peritoneum. The peritoneum is like a thin skin covering all the abdominal organs, and it ensures that they can move freely.

The esophagus, the stomach, and the intestine are made up of a muscular tube that is lined on the inside with a mucous membrane and covered on the outside by the peritoneum. Food is actively transported along this tube as a result of a rhythmic contraction of the muscles (peristalsis).

In the case of infection or inflammation, the process of regular, wavelike contractions is disturbed. This causes partially digested food to build up, gas to develop, and the intestinal wall to stretch. The irritation to the peritoneum results in cramplike pains. Severe contraction pains in the abdominal area are referred to as colic, and these occur most commonly as a result of irritation to the gallbladder or the urinary tract (gallstones and so forth).

Because the intestinal wall is only a few millimeters thick, if it is stretched inflammatory processes can go beyond it and spread throughout the abdomen. This is particularly dangerous in the case of acute appendicitis.

Symptoms

- Cramplike pains that can occur in different places
- Nausea and vomiting as evidence of impaired peristalsis
- Diarrhea as an indication of accelerated transport of food or of the intestine's inability to absorb water
- Fever as a sign of extensive inflammation

Treatment Guidelines

- No solid foods
- Plenty of fluids in the form of tea, mineral water, clear soup
- Damp body compresses
- Lowering of fever, possibly localized cooling
- Antispasmodic remedies:
  Plant-based: celandine, uzara, bitters, chamomile
  Chemical: N-butylscopalamine, trospiumchloride, metamizole

Important!

Antispasmodic remedies, including plant-based ones, can leave the impression that the condition has improved and conceal important symptoms—for instance, in the case of appendicitis.

Dosage instructions for children must be followed at all times. Overdoses can lead to a breakdown of intestinal activity.

A cooling treatment is advisable for illnesses with a high degree of inflammation.

For people with a history of heart disease, nausea and cramplike pains in the upper abdomen may indicate a heart attack.

ABDOMINAL CRAMPS

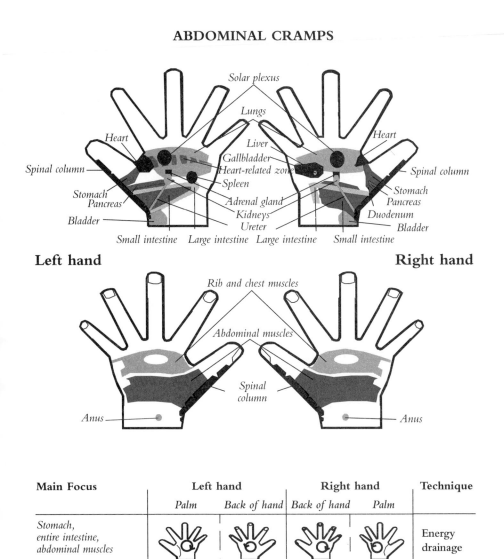

Left hand

Right hand

Main Focus	Left hand		Right hand		Technique
	Palm	Back of hand	Back of hand	Palm	
Stomach, entire intestine, abdominal muscles					Energy drainage
—					Energy buildup

3.2 Bile duct disorders

Definition

Bile serves the liver as a medium for excreting toxins. It also plays an important role in the digestion of fat. The bile ducts of the liver all come together in an excretory duct, which usually opens together with the pancreas exit duct into the duodenum. The opening is shaped like a button and has a sphincter that ensures the release of the right amount of digestive juices to the chyme. To the side of the bile duct is the gallbladder that serves as a reservoir for the bile.

These are some of the most common conditions affecting the bile ducts:
- Infection of the bile ducts due to pathogens
- Formation of gallstones causing inflammation and a shift of the bile ducts
- Functional disorder of the gallbladder
- Tumors in the bile ducts
- Mechanical shifting of the bile ducts from the outside

Symptoms

Bile duct inflammation leads to:
- Pain in the upper abdomen
- Fever, increase in white blood cells

If there is a shift of bile ducts, the bile cannot drain properly, resulting in:
- Convulsions of the bile ducts (colic)
- Reflux of bile pigments and their absorption by the blood
- Excretion of bile pigments via the urine (dark discoloration)
- Deposit of bile pigments in the tissue (icterus)

Treatment Guidelines

Treatment depends on the causes, which can generally be determined with simple, low-impact examinations.

In the case of minor complaints, it is helpful to treat the symptoms:
- Controlled intake of fats and proteins in the diet
- Damp body compresses as an antispasmodic remedy
- Medications:
  Plant-based: celandine, peppermint, turmeric, wormwood, dandelion
  Chemical: N-butylscopalamine, trospiumchloride, hymecromon

Important!
Severe inflammation of the bile ducts is a very serious condition and needs to be treated by a doctor. Rapid treatment with anti-inflammatory drugs and antibiotics, as well as surgical measures, are often essential and can save the patient's life.

BILE DUCT DISORDERS

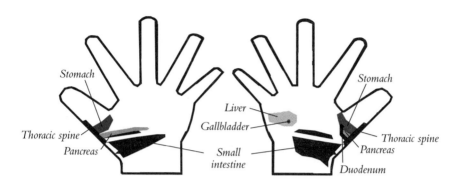

Left hand   **Right hand**

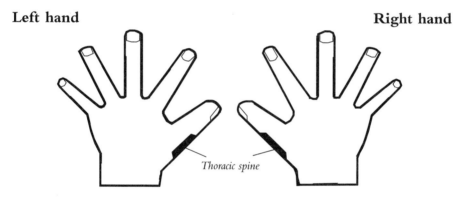

Main Focus	Left hand		Right hand		Technique
	Palm	Back of hand	Back of hand	Palm	
Gallbladder, liver, stomach					Energy drainage
——					Energy buildup

3.3 Constipation

Definition

Constipation refers to a malfunction of the intestine in which the transport of chyme is slowed down. Because the chyme remains in the large intestine for longer than normal, water is lost, causing excessively hard stools. Transport along the rectum and eventual evacuation can be severely impaired, and are no longer possible without help.

The causes of this widespread condition can be found mainly in an improper diet and poor habits:

- Not enough fiber in the diet
- Insufficient fluid intake
- Lack of exercise
- Regular use of laxatives, including plant-based remedies

Symptoms

Constipation often results in:

- Sensation of pressure in the upper abdomen
- Tendency toward flatulence
- Problems with bowel movements
- Formation of hemorrhoids
- Cramping or tearing of the anal sphincter

Experts are increasingly convinced today that an improper diet and subsequent constipation can cause intestinal tumors to develop.

Treatment Guidelines

The main objective is a sensible diet, but opinions are divided on this subject. The following basic rules, however, should be adhered to:

- Food should be high in fiber (whole-grain products, raw fruit and vegetables).
- The daily intake of fluids should be adjusted accordingly.
- Nicotine, caffeine, alcohol, and sugar intake should be eliminated completely or reduced to a minimum.
- Sufficient exercise is necessary over the course of the day.
- Laxatives should be used only sporadically, but are best avoided altogether.

Important!

Frequent use of laxatives (even plant-based products) damages the intestinal wall and significantly increases the risk of cancer!

Weight-loss diets are not a sensible way to eat, because, in the long run, they mean a one-sided diet causing nutrient deficiencies.

Unusual stools or blood in the stool may indicate a serious bowel disorder and should be examined by a doctor.

CONSTIPATION

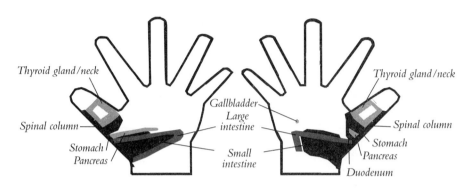

Thyroid gland/neck
Spinal column
Stomach
Pancreas
Gallbladder
Large intestine
Small intestine
Thyroid gland/neck
Spinal column
Stomach
Pancreas
Duodenum

Left hand   **Right hand**

Spinal column
Anus

Main Focus	Left hand		Right hand		Technique
	Palm	*Back of hand*	*Back of hand*	*Palm*	
Large intestine					Energy drainage
———					Energy buildup

3.4 Diarrhea

Definition

Diarrhea refers to an evacuation of loose-to-liquid stools, often in conjunction with an increased need to open the bowels. The causes are impaired water reabsorption from the chyme in the large intestine and accelerated transport of the chyme along the whole intestine. This is often due to:
- Pathogens (viruses, bacteria, fungi)
- Toxins
- Inflammation of the intestine (Crohn's disease, ulcerative colitis, diverticulitis)
- Stress (irritable bowel syndrome)

Not only is diarrhea a hygiene problem, but it also causes the body to lose valuable minerals and water.

Symptoms

- Loose-to-liquid stools
- More frequent bowel movements
- Unpleasant urge to open one's bowels
- Cramplike pain, especially when emptying one's bowels
- Weakened circulation due to loss of minerals and fluid

Treatment Guidelines

- Replace fluids and minerals.
- If symptoms persist, take calming and anti-inflammatory remedies, such as:
  Plant-based: chamomile, coal, bulk materials (apple pectin)
  Chemical: metoclopramide, loperamide
  Biological: milieu sanitation of the intestinal flora (E-coli fractions, saccharomyces cultures)

Important!
Loss of fluids and minerals is particularly dangerous for children and the elderly.

During the first 24 hours, the only treatment should be to replace fluids. Medication becomes necessary only if there has been an extreme loss of fluids.

Chronic diarrhea should be examined by a doctor to rule out causes such as salmonella.

DIARRHEA

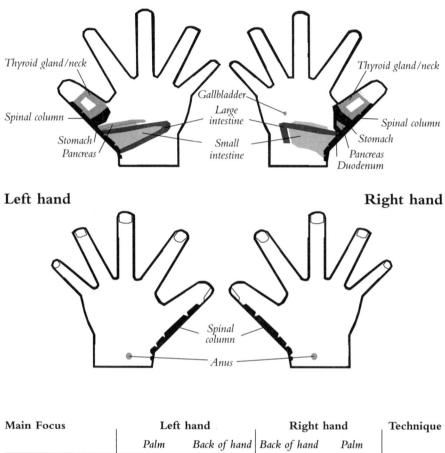

Left hand **Right hand**

Main Focus	Left hand		Right hand		Technique
	Palm	*Back of hand*	*Back of hand*	*Palm*	
Entire intestine					Energy drainage
Large intestine, anus					Energy buildup

3.5 Flatulence

Definition

Flatulence describes an accumulation of gases in the interior of the intestine. It can be caused by fermentation or by impaired gas absorption through the intestinal wall. Certain foods such as cabbage can cause an excessive production of gases in their digestion that the intestinal wall is temporarily unable to absorb. Flatulence complaints usually disappear within a short period of time and do not require treatment. However, this is a different matter with chronic fermentation and putrefaction processes in the intestine, which are often caused by:

- An improper diet
- Insufficient chewing of food
- Disturbed transportation of food
- Insufficient proportion of gastric juices from the stomach, the gallbladder, and the pancreas
- Disturbed intestinal flora (unfavorable bacteria settling in the intestine)

Symptoms

- Feeling of fullness, often two to three hours after meals
- Increased girth
- Cramplike, wandering abdominal pain
- Gurgling peristaltic sounds
- Foul-smelling anal gas emissions

Treatment Guidelines

In addition to an improved diet that includes plenty of fiber, it may be useful to:

- Take your time over meals, and chew your food thoroughly.
- Drink sufficient fluids.
- Exercise, especially after meals.

Depending on the symptoms, the condition can be treated with these medications:

- Plant-based: bitters such as wormwood, gentian, bitter orange, sweet flag *(Acorus calamus)*; carminatives and digestives such as fennel, caraway, aniseed, ginger, peppermint, melissa
- Chemical: dimeticon

Important!
If problems persist despite changes in diet and eating habits, a doctor should be consulted to rule out intestinal diseases and metabolic disorders.

FLATULENCE

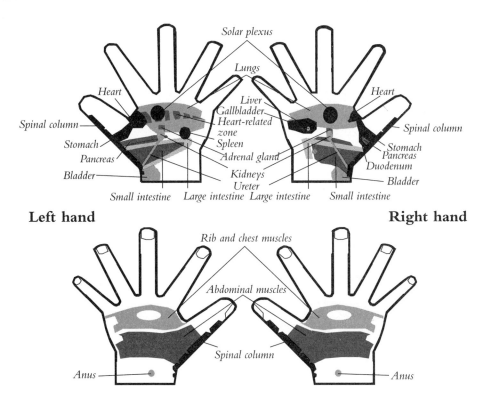

Left hand   **Right hand**

Main Focus	Left hand		Right hand		Technique
	Palm	Back of hand	Back of hand	Palm	
Entire intestine, abdominal muscles	🖐	🖐	🖐	🖐	Energy drainage
——	🖐	🖐	🖐	🖐	Energy buildup

3.6 Heartburn

Definition

Heartburn describes an irritation of the lower esophagus caused by gastric acid as a result of:

- A disturbed digestive process
- Increased production of gastric acid
- Impaired sphincter function at the entrance to the stomach—for instance, due to a diaphragmatic hernia

The esophagus runs inside the ribcage and opens into the stomach shortly after passing through the diaphragm. Because it joins up at the side of the stomach and there is a ring of muscles at the joint, the entrance to the stomach is usually sealed off very effectively, preventing the reflux of gastric acid into the esophagus. Unlike the stomach, the esophagus is not equipped with a mucous membrane, so any contact with gastric acid results in burning pain and convulsions. Prolonged contact with acid burns the wall of the esophagus, and the formation of scars during the healing process can lead to its narrowing.

In the case of a diaphragmatic hernia, the stomach entrance often slides through the enlarged opening in the diaphragm and the seal is no longer effective.

If the digestive process is disturbed, this is usually a result of poor eating habits.

Symptoms

- Heartburn is experienced as a burning pain in the upper abdomen and behind the sternum.
- It often occurs after large meals eaten too quickly.
- It frequently causes problems when lying down immediately after a meal.

Treatment Guidelines

The main objective is the normalization of eating habits:

- Eat several small meals a day.
- Eat slowly.
- Chew your food well.
- Ensure a good balance of fats and proteins in your diet.
- Avoid lying down after meals.

With acute complaints, depending on the severity of the problem, the following remedies can be helpful:

- Plant-based: liquorice, carminatives, bitters
- Chemical: acid buffers (aluminum hydroxide preparations), acid inhibitors (such as H2-blockers), remedies that strengthen the stomach wall (metoclopramide, cisapride)

Important!
Before you even consider medical treatment, you need to change your eating habits. The first time the problem occurs, or if it persists over a period of time, it's important to consult your doctor.

HEARTBURN

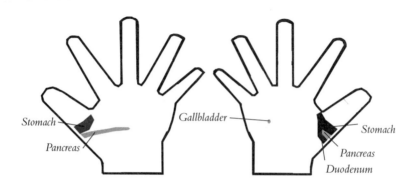

Stomach

Pancreas

Gallbladder

Stomach

Pancreas

Duodenum

Left hand **Right hand**

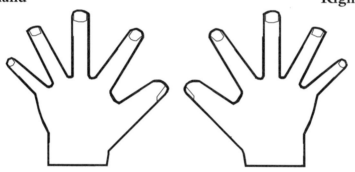

Main Focus	Left hand		Right hand		Technique
	Palm	*Back of hand*	*Back of hand*	*Palm*	
Stomach	🖐	🖐	🖐	🖐	Energy drainage
——	🖐	🖐	🖐	🖐	Energy buildup

3.7 Hemorrhoids

Definition

Hemorrhoids develop as the veins in the anal lining expand due to an increase in pressure in the blood vessels. This is caused by a raised blood supply via the arteries, impaired drainage from the veins, and reduced resistance of the tissue surrounding the blood vessels—conditions similar to those for varicose veins in the legs.

Apart from a genetic predisposition, the causes of this modern-day disorder can be found in behavioral patterns that can easily be avoided. The development of hemorrhoids is encouraged by:
- Working in a predominantly sedentary position
- Lack of exercise
- Low-fiber diet
- Chronic constipation

These factors mechanically impede the draining of blood from the anal veins. In addition, the pressure in the blood vessels rises severely if a lot of pressure is used to evacuate the bowels, and the intestinal wall is overly stretched and cannot support the blood vessels very well.

Symptoms

These are some of the initial signs pointing to the development of hemorrhoids:
- Itching and inflammation of the anus
- Burning sensation with each bowel movement
- Discharge from the anus

Symptoms occurring in the later stages of the condition include the following:
- Unpleasant urge to move one's bowels and painful evacuations
- Blood on the stools
- Impaired sphincter function

Treatment Guidelines

Medications and other therapeutic measures alone do not suffice; it is necessary to change your lifestyle. A sensible diet, sufficient exercise, and avoiding long periods of sitting can remove the causes of the condition and make any further symptom-relieving therapy redundant.

Various plant-based and chemical anti-inflammatory preparations can be used in the form of creams or suppositories. In severe cases, often the only option is surgery.

Important!
If you notice an anal discharge containing blood or mucus, your doctor should examine you to determine whether or not this may be caused by a tumor. Only if a tumor has been ruled out can you be sure that the diagnosis is really hemorrhoids.

HEMORRHOIDS

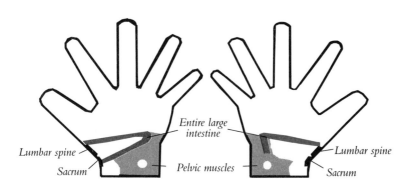

Left hand   **Right hand**

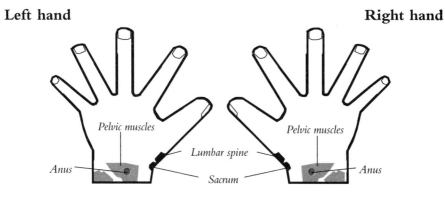

Main Focus	Left hand		Right hand		Technique
	Palm	*Back of hand*	*Back of hand*	*Palm*	
Large intestine, anus					Energy drainage
———					Energy buildup

3.8 Liver disorders

Definition

The liver is the main metabolic organ in the body. All draining blood vessels from the stomach-and-intestinal area come together in the portal circulation and open into the liver. There, the blood, which is full of nutrients and toxins, is filtered for the first time. From the liver, it flows back via the vena cava to the main blood circulation system. In the liver, nutrients are processed and stored so that they can be released back into the bloodstream when needed. Toxins can be excreted directly from the liver via bile, or they can be chemically altered so that they can be excreted by means of the kidneys.

Liver pain develops because the liver capsule becomes stretched—for example, from an inflammatory swelling. Infections with pathogens (particularly viruses) or strain from alcohol, poisons, medications, or overeating can cause inflammatory swelling. Severe inflammation can lead to scarring of the liver tissue, which results in the loss of its detoxifying function (cirrhosis of the liver).

Another common problem is impaired drainage of bile caused by the formation of stones in the bile ducts. The buildup of bile leads to bile pigment passing into the bloodstream, resulting in the body turning yellow in color (known as icterus).

Symptoms

- Sensation of pressure and pain on the right side of the upper abdomen
- Colic during the passing of gallstones into the bile ducts
- Exhaustion, tiredness, reduced performance
- Yellowing of the skin, also of the whites of the eyes (sclerenicterus)
- Darkening of urine

Treatment Guidelines

Before treatment begins, an exact diagnosis must be made. This is usually possible through simple examinations such as feeling the liver, ultrasound scans, or blood tests. Treatment then depends on the exact condition, although the following guidelines can be useful for anyone:

- Avoid unnecessary strain on the liver—for example, toxins, certain foods, alcohol, nicotine.
- Get plenty of rest.
- Unfortunately, there is no special "liver diet."

Important!
Liver diseases contracted during or after travel to exotic places should be examined immediately, as conditions caused by pathogens can often be treated successfully only in their early stages.

A fatty liver should not be taken lightly, because overeating, excessive alcohol consumption, and permanent strain due to toxins can lead to a chronic inflammation at first and then to the dangerous cirrhosis of the liver.

LIVER DISORDERS

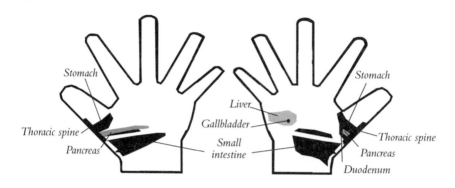

Left hand

Right hand

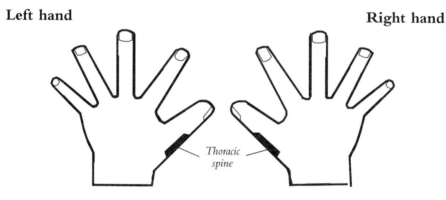

Main Focus	Left hand		Right hand		Technique
	Palm	Back of hand	Back of hand	Palm	
Gallbladder, liver					Energy drainage
———					Energy buildup

3.9 Pancreas complaints

Definition

The pancreas fulfills two main tasks with regard to digestion and metabolism. It produces enzymes that break down fats and proteins, which pass through an excretory duct into the duodenum. As a rule, the pancreas exit duct and the bile duct jointly open into the duodenum, resulting in the possibility that diseases in this area can affect several organs at the same time. Inflammatory processes are the most common, and they can progress very dramatically and be quite painful. Inflammation is frequently due to obstructions such as gallstones or tumors, infections caused by pathogens, or damage resulting from toxins like alcohol. The pancreatic islet cells produce the hormone insulin that transports blood sugar into the body's cells. If there is an imbalance in this area, it can often go unnoticed for a long time because it isn't accompanied by pain. The condition becomes evident only if there is a significant imbalance in the sugar metabolism.

Symptoms

- Inflammation of the pancreas causes a belt of pain circling the body at navel level.
- Insufficient production of digestive enzymes will cause flatulence and digestive problems.

An insulin imbalance is often characterized by:

- Tiredness, exhaustion, weight loss
- Increased thirst and frequency of urination
- Circulatory reactions, cold sweats

Treatment Guidelines

With inflammatory conditions of the pancreas, treatment must initially focus on their causes, such as the removal of obstructive gallstones. In addition, the following general measures are beneficial:

- Small meals with a balanced fat-and-protein content
- Enzyme preparations with a high content of pancreatic enzymes
- Rest

If an insulin imbalance is present, treatment depends on its severity:

- Normalization of body weight
- Controlled intake of carbohydrates (such as sugar, starch, potatoes, rice)
- Medications to improve the release of insulin (for example, glibenclamide)
- Insulin treatment

Important!
Diseases of the pancreas should always be taken very seriously and should initially be treated by a doctor. Alcohol and a poor diet are among the most common causes and must be avoided immediately. Regular checkups will help to diagnose conditions like diabetes at the start.

PANCREAS COMPLAINTS

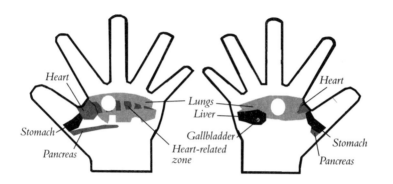

Heart

Lungs
Liver

Heart

Stomach

Gallbladder
Heart-related
zone

Stomach

Pancreas

Pancreas

Left hand

Right hand

Main Focus	Left hand		Right hand		Technique
	Palm	Back of hand	Back of hand	Palm	
Pancreas, heart					Energy drainage
——					Energy buildup

3.10 Stomach pain

The stomach is the continuation of the esophagus, just below the diaphragm. Food is mixed with gastric acid in the stomach not only to process the food but also to kill the majority of pathogens. The stomach wall itself is protected from the effects of gastric acid by a thick mucous lining. If this lining is weakened or if acid production is very high, the stomach wall becomes irritated and painful. However, an excessive mechanical stretching of the stomach can cause pains similar to cramps in the upper abdomen. If the stomach wall becomes inflamed as a result of constant irritation, this is referred to as gastritis. When the inflammation spreads, the mucous lining breaks open, leading to the formation of deep, crater-shaped wounds called stomach ulcers. The following factors encourage the development of inflammatory disorders of the stomach wall:

- A high-fat and high-protein diet, eating too quickly
- Stress
- Excessive consumption of nicotine and alcohol

Symptoms

- Burning, stabbing, or cramplike pains at the center of the upper abdomen
- Hunger pains
- Feeling of fullness, heartburn after meals
- Black discoloration of stools

Treatment Guidelines

The condition can often be improved by simply adjusting your eating habits. Prior to a course of medication, you should try the measures below:

- Reducing your alcohol and nicotine intake
- Avoiding foods that are high in fat and proteins
- Eating several small meals instead of a few large ones
- Relaxing and exercising sufficiently
- Medications:
  Plant-based: bitters, cinchona bark, gentian, peppermint, caraway, melissa, wormwood
  Chemical: acid buffers (antacids, usually magnesium salts), acid inhibitors (for example, ranitidine, cimetidine, omeprazol), strengthening remedies (for example, metoclopramide, cisapride)

Important!
If stomach pains persist for more than two weeks despite sensible therapy, they should be examined by a doctor. A gastroscopy is not a pleasant procedure, but it can often prevent much more unpleasant emergency measures.

Black stools are a symptom of bleeding in the stomach or the duodenum and need to be examined right away. Stomach cancer is one of the most common cancers, but unfortunately is often recognized too late.

STOMACH PAIN

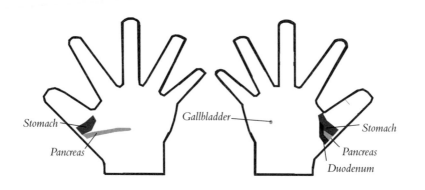

Left hand

Right hand

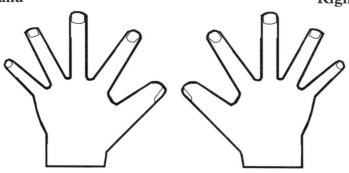

Main Focus	Left hand		Right hand		Technique
	Palm	Back of hand	Back of hand	Palm	
Stomach					Energy drainage
——					Energy buildup

4. Urinary and Sexual Organs

4.1 Bladder complaints

4.2 Disorders of the ovaries and fallopian tubes

4.3 Disorders of the uterus

4.4 Female infertility

4.5 Kidney disorders

4.6 Male impotence

4.7 Mammary gland disorders

4.8 Menopausal problems

4.9 Menstrual problems

4.10 Problems during pregnancy

4.11 Prostate complaints

4.1 Bladder complaints

Definition

The bladder receives urine from the kidneys via two ureters. It is a very elastic muscle sack that is lined on the inside by a thick mucous membrane to protect it against the aggressive urine. The bladder is emptied via the urethra. In women, this is only a few centimeters long and opens into the anterior vagina. In men, however, the urethra runs through the prostate gland, where the seminal ducts join, and on through the entire penis.

The emptying of the bladder is a complicated process, controlled by:

- Pressure that indicates that the bladder is full
- Active contractions of the bladder wall
- Straightening of the urethra by lifting the pelvic floor
- Relaxation of a loop-shaped sphincter at the bladder exit

The most common bladder complaints in women are infections with pathogens and impaired sealing function (incontinence) as a result of a lowering of the sexual organs. In men, drainage problems because of a swollen prostate are more common.

Symptoms

- Pain in the central lower abdomen
- Burning sensation while passing water or afterward
- Aches radiating into the loins
- Urge to urinate
- Spontaneous urination or dripping, especially caused by coughing, pushing, sitting, and walking

Treatment Guidelines

Treatment depends on the cause of the condition. A urine sample can be tested for infections or inflammation. In either case, the following measures will always be beneficial:

- Increased fluid intake, about 2 to 3 quarts, or liters, a day
- Cold, damp compresses against pain
- Anti-inflammatory, antispasmodic medications:
  Chemical: acetylsalicylic acid, diclofenac, N-butylscopalamine
  Plant-based: bearberry, birch tree leaves, echinacea, saw palmetto
  Antibiotics: a doctor's prescription of trimethoprim, sulfamethoxazol, gyrase inhibitors, for example, if pathogens have been found

---

Important!
Blood in the urine may indicate a tumor in the bladder, and should be examined if this occurs frequently or over a period of time.

BLADDER COMPLAINTS

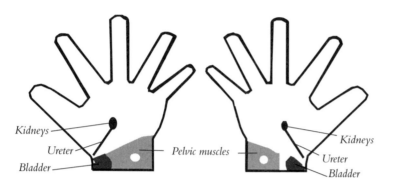

Kidneys
Ureter
Bladder
Pelvic muscles
Kidneys
Ureter
Bladder

Left hand   **Right hand**

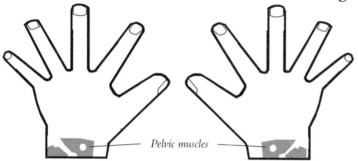

Pelvic muscles

Main Focus	Left hand		Right hand		Technique
	Palm	Back of hand	Back of hand	Palm	
Bladder	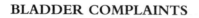				Energy drainage
———					Energy buildup

4.2 Disorders of the ovaries and fallopian tubes

Definition

The ovaries (from the Latin *ovum,* meaning "egg") contain the female germ cells. Under the cyclical influence of the sexual hormones, individual ova mature in the ovaries until they are ready to be fertilized. Halfway through the cycle, one egg is usually expelled from a mature follicle into the abdominal cavity and travels along the fallopian tube to the uterus. Fertilization by a semen cell takes place while the egg is still in the fallopian tube. The fertilized egg then implants itself in the lining of the uterus, where it continues its development.

Common disorders relating to the ovaries and fallopian tubes include the following:
- Hormonally influenced changes such as a disturbed maturing of follicles
- Inflammation and bleeding during ovulation
- Infections due to pathogens
- Planting of the fertilized egg outside the uterus
- Formation of fluid-filled caverns (cysts)
- Tumors

Symptoms

Inflammation of the ovaries causes these symptoms:
- Lower abdominal pain
- Fever (frequently)

Tumors or cysts cause these:
- Sensation of pressure
- Increased girth

Treatment Guidelines

Inflammations should be inhibited quickly to prevent them from spreading throughout the pelvis. Here are some useful measures:
- Cooling compresses
- Anti-inflammatory medications (such as diclofenac, naproxen, ibuprofen)
- If necessary, antibiotics

With problems having to do with the menstrual cycle, hormonal imbalances should be considered initially. If symptoms are mild and short-lived, treatment is not always necessary. Inflammation and scarring of the fallopian tubes may present obstacles for eggs and can frequently be the reason why a woman does not become pregnant. The ovaries themselves produce sexual hormones that not only play an important role during early pregnancy but also in bringing about a normal menstrual cycle.

> **Important!**
> Pain and symptoms of inflammation in the lower abdomen can be caused by any of the abdominal organs, and therefore require a detailed examination to determine the exact cause. If the pain is localized on the right side of the lower abdomen, be sure that you are checked for appendicitis.

DISORDERS OF THE OVARIES AND FALLOPIAN TUBES

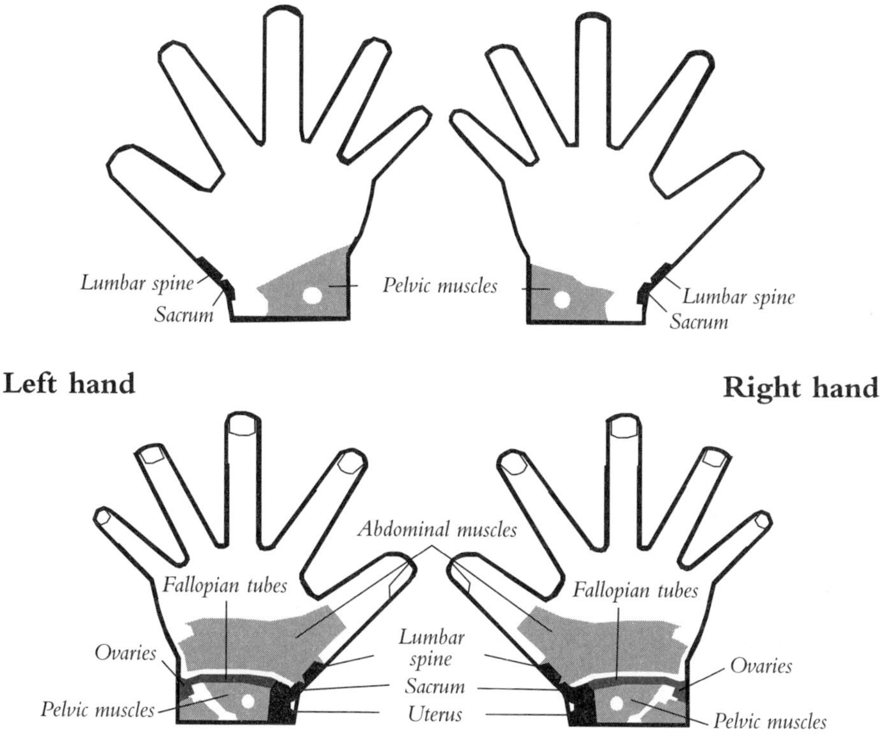

Lumbar spine
Sacrum
Pelvic muscles
Lumbar spine
Sacrum

Left hand

Right hand

Abdominal muscles
Fallopian tubes
Fallopian tubes
Ovaries
Lumbar spine
Sacrum
Ovaries
Pelvic muscles
Uterus
Pelvic muscles

Main Focus	Left hand		Right hand		Technique
	Palm	Back of hand	Back of hand	Palm	
Ovaries, fallopian tubes	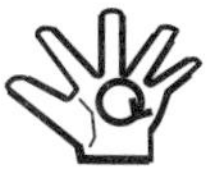	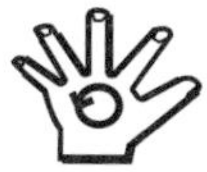	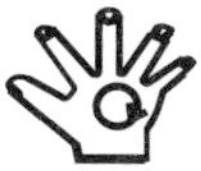	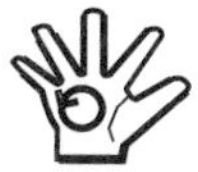	Energy drainage
———	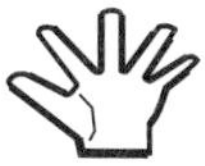	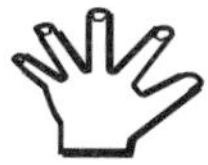	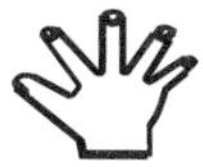	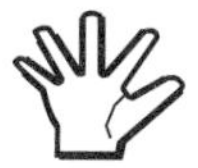	Energy buildup

4.3 Disorders of the uterus

Definition

The uterus has a muscle wall and is lined on the inside with a mucous membrane. The membrane changes under the cyclical influence of hormones. Some of the female sexual hormones, the estrogens, cause the uterus lining to increase in size and thicken. At the end of the cycle, menstrual bleeding takes place as the lining is expelled from the uterus and travels by way of the cervix into the vagina.

Common disorders of the uterus include the following:
- Impaired formation of the mucous membrane
- Inflammation or infection
- Premature or incomplete detachment of the mucous membrane
- Tumors in the muscle wall (usually benign, as with myoma)

Symptoms

Infections and inflammation are accompanied by:
- Pain in the central lower abdomen

However, hormone-related problems are more frequent:
- Premature withdrawal bleeding
- Heavier menstrual bleeding than normal
- Bleeding between menstrual periods

Treatment Guidelines

Problems related to the menstrual cycle can be treated with:
- Natural and synthetic hormones

Inflammation and infections are treated with:
- Anti-inflammatory medications
- Antibiotics

If the uterus becomes enlarged as a result of tumors, they will need to be removed surgically.

Important!
With increasing age, there is a growing risk of tumors forming in the uterus, especially around the cervix.

DISORDERS OF THE UTERUS

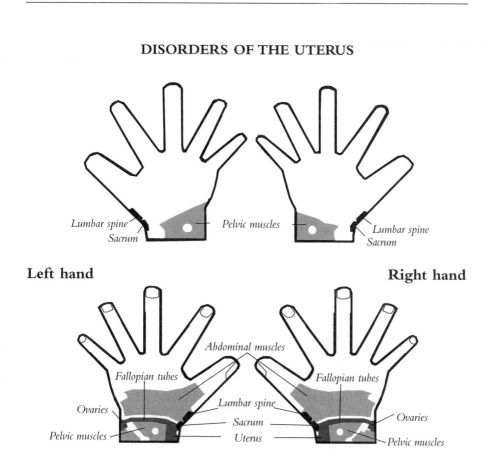

Left hand

Right hand

Main Focus	Left hand		Right hand		Technique
	Palm	*Back of hand*	*Back of hand*	*Palm*	
Ovaries, fallopian tubes, uterus					Energy drainage
———					Energy buildup

4.4 Female infertility

Definition

Infertility in women means the inability of a woman to become pregnant despite the desire to have children or to carry a baby successfully to term. Causes may include the following:
- Disorders of the ovaries, fallopian tubes, uterus, or hormonal glands
- Impaired function of otherwise healthy organs—for instance, as a result of stress

In order for a woman to become pregnant and carry the baby to term, a multitude of factors must be met:
- Normal maturing of healthy ova in the ovaries
- Normal ovulation
- Fertilization of the ovum at the right time and place
- Preparation of the mucous membrane of the uterus
- The fertilized egg's being implanted in the lining of the uterus
- Development of the placenta, the link to the mother's blood circulation
- Undisturbed development of the baby
- Onset of the birth process at the right time

Symptoms

In today's society, where such a high premium is placed on success, being unable to have a child despite wanting one becomes a serious problem for many couples. Although the causes are frequently unknown, women are still commonly blamed for this situation, often experiencing the following:
- Feelings of inferiority
- Fear of failure
- Depression
- Stress

Treatment Guidelines

In the past, even if a disease had been diagnosed, the chances of a successful pregnancy were often merely reduced. However, today, not only can many conditions be diagnosed, but their causes can also be treated. Frequently, such problems are of a psycho-vegetative nature, either exclusively or in addition to an existing disease. Of course, if these problems are related to a woman's psyche, environmental influences, stress at work, or to her relationship with her partner, surgical measures or treatment with medicines will not bring the desired result. In such cases, there are other helpful measures, including:
- Stress management
- Resolving conflicts in the relationship

> **Important!**
> Trying to have a child at all costs is problematic. Make sure that you are aware of all the possible risks involved. The best technological methods cannot overcome psychological barriers.

FEMALE INFERTILITY

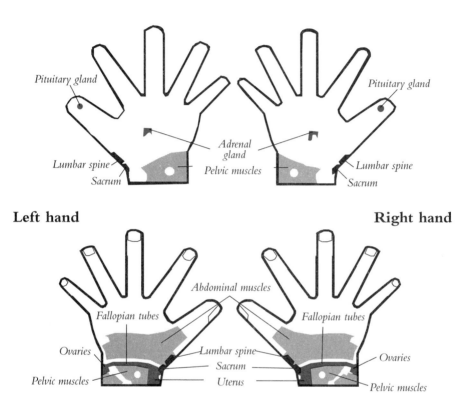

Left hand **Right hand**

Main Focus	Left hand		Right hand		Technique
	Palm	Back of hand	Back of hand	Palm	
All abdominal organs, adrenal gland, pituitary gland, thyroid gland/ neck					Energy drainage
———					Energy buildup

4.5 Kidney disorders

Definition

The kidneys are important organs that deal with excretions and regulate the body's mineral-and-water balance. In the kidneys, the solid and liquid constituents of the blood are separated and, while the liquid constituent leaves the kidneys, the solid constituents such as blood cells and large protein particles remain behind in the kidneys' blood vessels. The fluid that leaves the kidneys not only contains toxins but also essential minerals, proteins, and water. Following the countercurrent principle, these substances can be reabsorbed from the excreted liquid through a complicated pipe network using little energy. In order to do their work, the kidneys depend on as regular a circulatory pressure as possible. They therefore produce specific hormones that play an important role in regulating blood pressure and constitute an important factor in the circulatory system.

Common kidney disorders include the following:

● Rising infections from the bladder, caused by pathogens
● Impaired drainage—for example, due to kidney stones
● Diminished detoxifying function, weakened kidneys

Symptoms

The following complaints are typical of kidney disorders:

■ Aches down the side of the body and in the back
■ Colic (contraction pains coming in waves)

Many disorders, however, don't display any noticeable symptoms, and can often be diagnosed only by changes in the urine:

■ Foaming (high protein content)—nephritis, kidney damage
■ Red coloring (urine contains blood)—kidney stones, nephritis
■ Clouding (protein, white blood cells)—nephritis, infections
■ Smell (acetone)—diabetes

Treatment Guidelines

Treatment must be preceded by an exact diagnosis of what is causing the complaint. For acute complaints but also as preventive measures, observe the guidelines below:

◆ Drink plenty of fluids.
◆ Avoid toxins that need to be excreted via the kidneys (uric acid, medications, poisons).
◆ Undergo correct treatment of metabolic disorders (such as diabetes).
◆ Get proper treatment for infections.

Important!
Many kidney disorders can slowly and without noticeable problems lead to permanent damage. As the kidneys increasingly fail to work properly, toxins are no longer excreted completely, upsetting the body's mineral-and-water balance.

KIDNEY DISORDERS

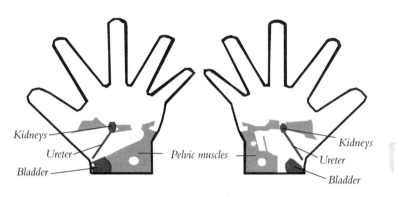

Kidneys — Ureter — Bladder — Pelvic muscles — Kidneys — Ureter — Bladder

Left hand **Right hand**

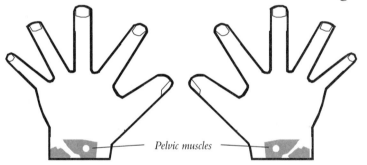

Pelvic muscles

Main Focus	Left hand		Right hand		Technique
	Palm	*Back of hand*	*Back of hand*	*Palm*	
Kidneys, ureter, bladder					Energy drainage
——					Energy buildup

4.6 Male impotence

Definition

Impotence is distinctly different from infertility. Infertility refers to the impossibility or reduced likelihood of fathering children, often caused by problems relating to sperm-cell formation. Impotence, on the other hand, pertains to problems with sexual intercourse. There can be a variety of causes:
- Physiological problems, especially with erections
- Lack of libido
- Psychological and social problems, such as conflicts between partners, personality-related problems, social stress

Symptoms

Sexuality is still somewhat of a taboo subject in our society. The natural drive to reproduce and preserve the species is an essential part of our being. Reproduction and sexual drive are closely linked to hierarchical orders and ambitions concerning power. If problems exist in these areas, men especially tend to deny them, as such problems could be regarded as a loss of personal power and social prestige. This conflict can result in:
- Fear of failure
- Feelings of inferiority
- Avoidance of problematic situations
- Aggression

Treatment Guidelines

It is often difficult to distinguish real physiological problems from the probably more common problems related to sexual drive and psychosocial issues. The symptoms are often the same, and the different areas are frequently related. The crux of the matter usually lies in the framework in which one's sexuality takes place. Thus, it's worth considering the following points:
- Problems with one's own personality (how do I see myself?)
- Problems regarding interacting with others (how do others see me?)
- Relationship problems (allocation of roles)
- Other factors (job, social environment, illness, and so forth)

When dealing with sensitive issues like impotence, it is important to assume as neutral a position as possible—something that is generally difficult for the person concerned, his partner, and the people in his immediate environment. For this reason, there are specialists who offer various forms of treatment, such as partner therapy, psychological counseling, and group therapy.

Important!
The use of sexual tonics or elixirs is problematic at best. Not only do they have a dubious effect, but with their use the real problem tends to be suppressed.

MALE IMPOTENCE

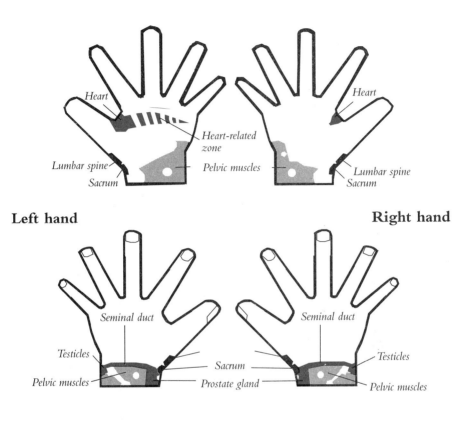

Left hand   **Right hand**

Main Focus	Left hand		Right hand		Technique
	Palm	*Back of hand*	*Back of hand*	*Palm*	
———					Energy drainage
Testicles, seminal duct, prostate gland, heart, heart-related zone					Energy buildup

4.7 Mammary gland disorders

Definition

Men and women have two mammary glands (in Latin, *mamma*; in Greek, *mastos*). Their exit ducts open into the nipples (mammillae). The female mammary glands are far more distinctive because of the influence of sexual hormones, and are characteristic of the outward appearance of women. In females, the mammary glands begin to develop during puberty as a result of hormonal changes and the reaching of sexual maturity. However, they continue to be susceptible to hormonal influences throughout life. When a woman has a baby, hormonal changes cause the mammary glands to produce and secrete milk, in order to feed the newborn.

Mammary gland disorders can occur as a result of:
- Hormonal imbalance, hormonal changes, hormone treatment
- Infections due to pathogens
- Scar formation in old age
- Tumors

Symptoms

Mastitis (inflammation of the mammary glands) is characterized by:
- Pain, swelling, reddening, breast feeling hot to the touch

Mastodynia (pain in the breast) is triggered by hormonal changes and results in:
- Aches and a sensation of pressure, dependent on the menstrual cycle

The mammillae are among the body's erogenous zones and become erect if they are stimulated. However, if they are stimulated too much, this can be painful. Symptoms of serious diseases of the mammary gland include the following:
- Secretions from the mammilla, especially if the secretion contains blood
- Increasingly hard mammary gland
- Enlarged lymph nodes under the arms

Treatment Guidelines

If the cause of the disorder lies outside the mammary gland itself, such as hormonal imbalance, that cause is what needs to be treated. Many of these disorders, however, are very temporary and short-lived, and treatment is therefore limited to the symptoms. Inflammation and infection should be treated immediately and efficiently:
- Inflammation can be brought down by cooling and with medications such as diclofenac, naproxen, or heparin cream.
- Antibiotics are another alternative.
- In the case of purulent caverns, surgical opening and draining is necessary.

Important!
Breast tumors are common and carry a high risk of becoming malignant. Therefore, it's wise to undergo regular checkups for your own safety and peace of mind.

MAMMARY GLAND DISORDERS

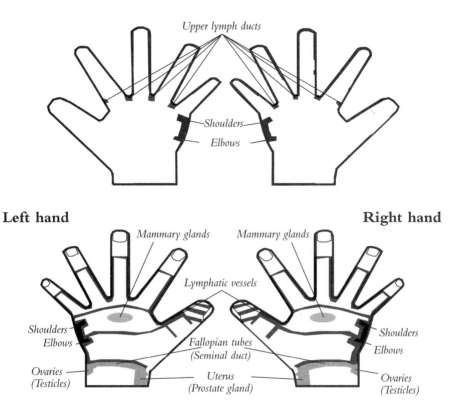

Upper lymph ducts

Shoulders
Elbows

Left hand   **Right hand**

Mammary glands   Mammary glands

Lymphatic vessels

Shoulders   Shoulders
Elbows   Elbows

Ovaries   Fallopian tubes
(Testicles)   (Seminal duct)
                 Uterus   Ovaries
                 (Prostate gland)   (Testicles)

Main Focus	Left hand		Right hand		Technique
	Palm	*Back of hand*	*Back of hand*	*Palm*	
Mammary glands, all lymphatic vessels					Energy drainage
———					Energy buildup

4.8 Menopausal problems

Definition

Around the age of 50, a woman's fertile years come to an end. This is a time characterized by hormonal changes, menopause. During this time, the ovaries produce less and less of the female sexual hormones, the estrogens. As the cycle of rhythmical hormone fluctuations is gradually weakened and eventually ceases to exist, women stop menstruating. Because the sexual hormones also influence regular functions in other organs, many women experience problems that require treatment. The following organs and areas are affected most severely:

- Sexual organs (mammary glands, ovaries, uterus, vagina)
- Bone metabolism (osteoporosis)
- Heart and circulatory system
- Autonomic nervous system (general organ control, metabolism)
- Psyche (moods, drive)

Symptoms

The signs of menopause can vary greatly and include the following:

- Irregular menstruation or continuous bleeding, prior to complete cessation of periods
- Vaginal dryness
- Vegetative symptoms:
  Hot flashes, cold shivers, sweats
  Palpitations, feeling of tightness in the chest and neck
  Sleeplessness, fear
  Overall reduction in performance, lack of drive
  Mood swings, depression, irritability
  Increase in risk factors (high blood pressure, impaired fat metabolism)
  Bones becoming brittle (osteoporosis)

Treatment Guidelines

For many years now, hormone-replacement therapy has been used to counterbalance the body's reduced production of its own hormones. Drawing on experience in this area, we would recommend the following:

- Start hormone-replacement therapy early on (in addition to alleviating the signs of menopause, it reduces the risk of heart and circulatory problems and of osteoporosis).
- If hormone preparations do not agree with you, or if you are opposed to using them for other reasons, try plant-based remedies that work in a similar way to hormones or have a balancing effect.
- Undergo calcitonin treatment if you are diagnosed as having osteoporosis (calcitonin is a hormone that improves calcium absorption by the bones).

Important!
During menopause, women run an increased risk of developing tumors in the sexual organs. Because of this, regular checkups are vital.

MENOPAUSAL PROBLEMS

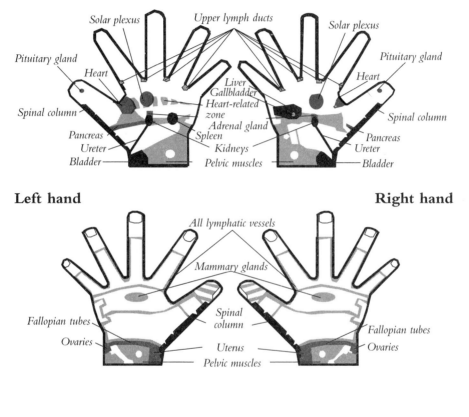

Left hand   **Right hand**

Main Focus	Left hand		Right hand		Technique
	Palm	Back of hand	Back of hand	Palm	
Pituitary gland, heart, solar plexus					Energy drainage
——					Energy buildup

4.9 Menstrual problems

Definition

Menstruation (from the Latin *menstruus,* meaning "monthly") refers to the cyclical changes affecting a woman's hormone balance. The duration of a cycle is approximately 28 days. During the first half of the cycle, a follicle containing an ovum matures in the ovaries (see 4.2, Disorders of the ovaries and fallopian tubes). While it is maturing, the follicle produces estrogens that result in the formation of the uterus lining. Following ovulation, the follicle is transformed into the corpus luteum and starts producing progesterone. Under the influence of progesterone, the lining of the uterus develops further and changes in order to be able to receive the ovum. If there is no implantation of a fertilized egg, the activity of the corpus luteum decreases. The highly developed uterus lining can no longer be sustained and is expelled in an inflammatory reaction, causing bleeding.

Symptoms

When the uterus lining is expelled, this may bring on:
- Lower abdominal pain
- A feeling of being physically unwell
- Vegetative symptoms such as nausea, circulatory problems, or headaches

Treatment Guidelines

Because the above complaints are only temporary and more or less short-lived, treatment should focus on only what is absolutely necessary. The following measures can be used to alleviate various menstrual problems:
- Relaxation techniques
- Damp body compresses
- Mild painkillers and vegetative remedies:
  Chemical: paracetamol, acetylsalicylic acid, propyphenazon/drofenine
  Plant-based: monk's pepper, arnica, calendula, chamomile, shepherd's purse, silverweed cinquefoil, cimicifuga root

---

Important!
Regular use of painkillers in high doses can lead to an increased sensitivity to pain and to addiction.

The body loses important nutrients, particularly iron, because of the blood loss. Therefore, women who have very heavy periods often suffer from anemia.

MENSTRUAL PROBLEMS

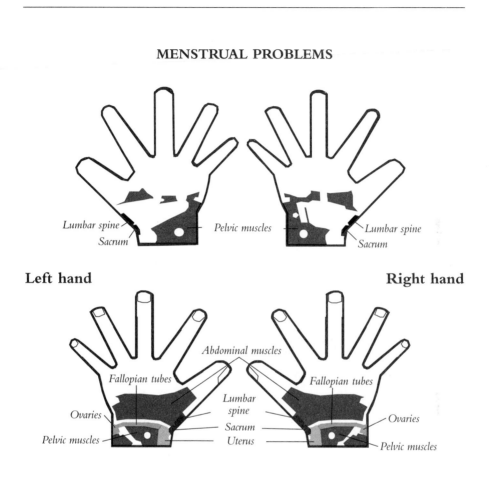

Lumbar spine
Sacrum
Pelvic muscles
Lumbar spine
Sacrum

Left hand

Right hand

Abdominal muscles
Fallopian tubes
Lumbar spine
Ovaries
Sacrum
Pelvic muscles
Uterus
Fallopian tubes
Ovaries
Pelvic muscles

Main Focus	Left hand		Right hand		Technique
	Palm	*Back of hand*	*Back of hand*	*Palm*	
Uterus, pelvic muscles, abdominal muscles					Energy drainage
———					Energy buildup

4.10 Problems during pregnancy

Definition

With problems during pregnancy, a clear distinction must be made between:
- Problems that occur during an otherwise normal pregnancy
- Problems that affect the pregnancy itself and carry a risk for both mother and child

It goes without saying that the latter always needs to be monitored and treated by a doctor, as this is the only way to keep the risk for mother and baby as low as possible during this critical period.

Complaints that occur during a normal pregnancy often cannot be treated with the usual means. This is particularly true when it comes to taking medications, which, when processed in the body, leave behind unknown waste products. It is impossible to assess what effect these waste products may have on a pregnant woman, and their formation depends on the situation and the individual. For this reason, medications should be used only if they are essential for the mother's well-being and there are no alternative measures available.

Symptoms

Common complaints during pregnancy include the following:
- Nausea, digestive problems
- Circulatory problems
- Overall drop in performance
- Problems affecting joints and the spine
- Mood swings

Treatment Guidelines

Many of these complaints occur only in bursts or for a short time. It is very rare that they need to be treated with medication. Prior to any medical treatment, try the measures below, if your doctor has established that they do not pose a risk to your pregnancy:
- For circulatory problems—endurance training in small doses
- For digestive problems—fresh, raw foods, plenty of fiber, exercise
- For overall drop in performance—planning your day, delegating tasks
- For problems affecting joints and the spine—exercises, especially for muscles
- For mood swings—physical activity and relaxation

There are many different ways to tackle these problems, but it takes some initiative to make use of them. It is often helpful if your partner takes an active interest as well.

Important!
Persistent complaints can often be treated with lower-risk plant-based alternatives to conventional medicines. However, even plant-based remedies can have side effects. Therefore, they should not be used during pregnancy without your doctor's consent.

PROBLEMS DURING PREGNANCY

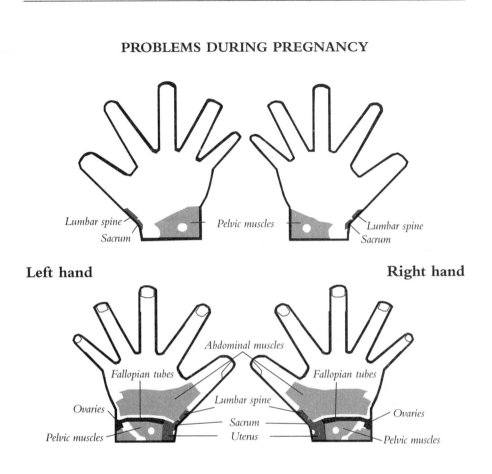

Left hand   **Right hand**

Main Focus	Left hand		Right hand		Technique
	Palm	Back of hand	Back of hand	Palm	
Uterus, sacrum, lumbar spine					Energy drainage
———					Energy buildup

4.11 Prostate complaints

Definition

In men, the prostate gland encircles the urethra immediately after it leaves the bladder. At this point, the seminal ducts join and open into the urethra. On ejaculation, a milky secretion is discharged from the prostate gland, which is vital for the function of the semen cells. Under the influence of sexual hormones, most men experience an enlargement of the prostate gland after the age of 50 (benign prostatic hypertrophy). This puts pressure on the urethra from the outside and causes it to narrow, making bladder evacuation more difficult. As with most hormone-dependent tissues, the prostate gland is severely at risk from malignant tumors (prostate carcinoma). In addition to age-related enlargement, inflammation of the prostate gland (prostatitis) is a common problem.

Symptoms

Prostate inflammation and enlargement usually lead to:
- Reduced pressure on the bladder and pain on evacuation (dysuria)
- Frequent urge to urinate
- Incomplete bladder evacuation (residual urine formation)
- Increased risk of infection of the urinary tract
- Pain on ejaculation

Treatment Guidelines

Treatment must start as early as possible. In addition to anti-inflammatory drugs and medications to treat infections, plant-based remedies are used to decrease the swelling. If these measures don't alleviate the complaint, there is also the option of surgery.
- Anti-inflammatory drugs:
  Chemical: diclofenac, ibuprofen
  Plant-based: saw palmetto, echinacea, bearberry, stinging nettle, horse chestnut
- Medications that inhibit growth:
  Plant-based: saw palmetto, pumpkin seeds, stinging nettle
- Surgical measures are carried out mainly with endoscopes (slim instruments) via the urethra.

Important!
About 20 to 30 percent of men over the age of 50 already show signs of developing a malignant prostate tumor, although they aren't experiencing any problems. Regular checkups are the only way to help recognize and treat this condition at the start. Yet only a small percentage of men actually take advantage of such checkups, either out of inertia or an unfounded sense of shame.

PROSTATE COMPLAINTS

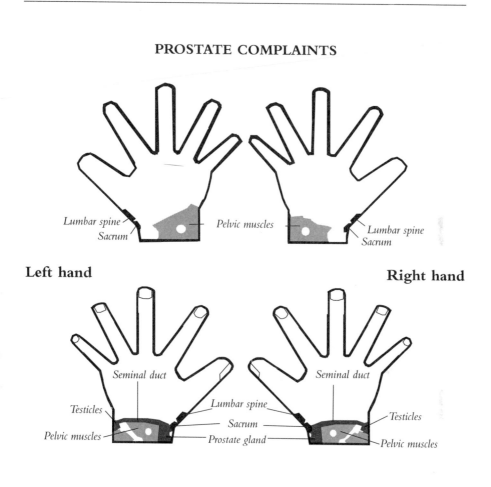

Lumbar spine
Sacrum
Pelvic muscles
Lumbar spine
Sacrum

Left hand

Right hand

Seminal duct
Seminal duct

Testicles
Lumbar spine
Testicles
Pelvic muscles
Sacrum
Pelvic muscles
Prostate gland

Main Focus	Left hand		Right hand		Technique
	Palm	Back of hand	Back of hand	Palm	
Testicles, seminal duct, prostate gland					Energy drainage
_____					Energy buildup

5. Spinal Column and Limbs

5.1 Complaints of the lower spinal column

5.2 Complaints of the upper spinal column

5.3 Disorders of the knee joint

5.4 Hip complaints

5.5 Injury aftercare

5.6 Muscular disorders

5.7 Rheumatic disorders

5.8 Shoulder pain

5.9 Tennis elbow

5.10 Varicose veins

5.1 Complaints of the lower spinal column

Definition

The lower spine comprises the lumbar vertebrae, the sacrum, and the coccyx. The spinal nerves of the lumbar vertebrae serve the legs. As with the cervical spine, they first form a plexus and then join up in the main nerves that supply the legs. The leg is primarily served by the sciatic nerve, which runs from the pelvis to the back and down the leg until it reaches the foot. The vertebrae of the sacrum have grown together to form a single bone, making mechanical irritation in this area quite rare. The coccyx does not play a role in keeping the body stable and causes problems only if it has suffered a direct injury. The lumbar spine, however, plays a significant role in keeping the body upright and stable. As it curves and is equipped with elastic disks, it has a similar function as the suspension of a car. The main movement that the lumbar spine carries out is bending forward from the hips, which is necessary for bending down and lifting.

Complaints of the lumbar spine are the most common:

- Localized pain around the lumbar spine (lumbago)
- Pain that radiates into a leg (ischialgia)
- A combination of both (lumbo-ischialgia)
- Prolapsed disk

Symptoms

These are the main symptoms of lumbar spine complaints:

- Pain, either localized or radiating into the legs
- Limited mobility
- Impaired sensation in the legs, legs feeling heavy
- Paralysis of the legs

Treatment Guidelines

The most common causes of problems with the lower spine are poor posture and incorrect weight distribution. Apart from dealing with the acute pain (see 5.2, Complaints of the upper spinal column), the following measures are beneficial:

- Normalization of weight
- Exercises to strengthen muscles
- Classes to improve posture
- Avoiding incorrect weight distribution:
  Bending over to lift something
  Sitting with a hollow-back or tense posture
  Compensatory measures if one leg is shorter than the other

Important!
Impaired sensation and loss of strength in the legs are signs of nerve damage. Nerve tissue is very sensitive and dies if it is persistently damaged. The longer such complaints remain untreated, the more unlikely it is that they will heal completely, without negative consequences.

COMPLAINTS OF THE LOWER SPINAL COLUMN

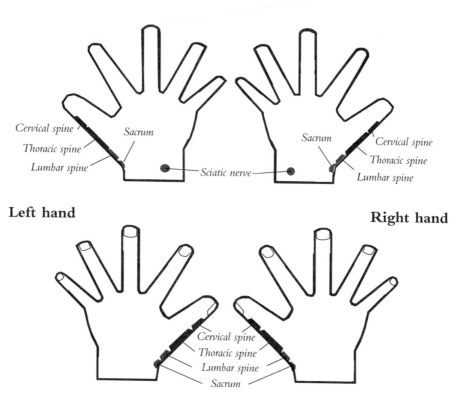

Left hand

Right hand

Main Focus	Left hand		Right hand		Technique
	Palm	Back of hand	Back of hand	Palm	
Lumbar spine, sacrum, sciatic nerve					Energy drainage
———					Energy buildup

5.2 Complaints of the upper spinal column

Definition

The cervical and thoracic spine form the upper section of the spinal column. The spinal nerves come out between the vertebral arches that are situated to the back. From the thoracic spine, the nerves run between the ribs and around the ribcage to the front, where they supply the skin, the subcutis, the muscles, and the ribs. From the cervical spine, nerves go out into the brachial plexus, from which three main nerves emerge to supply the arm.

Complaints of the upper spine are very common, and possible causes include the following:
- Mechanical irritation of emerging nerves
- Gaps between the vertebrae becoming smaller as the intervertebral disks wear down
- Bones and joints wearing down with age
- Inflammation of the surrounding soft parts

Symptoms

Complaints of the upper spine can occur close to the spine itself, but also along the nerve channels that are located in this area. These complaints manifest in a variety of ways:
- Limited ability to move the head, especially to turn it to the side
- Headaches that radiate from the back of the neck to the back of the head
- Shortening of the pectoral muscles, resulting in the shoulders' being hunched forward
- Tension in the rear shoulder muscles
- Limited ability to lift the arm up to the side

Treatment Guidelines

As the above are usually long-term and recurring problems, accompanied by inflammation and pain, the following measures may be useful:
- For quick pain relief and efficient abating of the inflammation:
  Medication: diclofenac, naproxen, piroxicam, ibuprofen
  Localized: neural therapy, wheal therapy, infiltrations, acupuncture
- For relaxation of tense muscles:
  Medication: chloromezanone, tetrazepam
  Mechanical: stretching, gymnastic exercises, massage
  Physical: heat (hot air, infrared lamp, microwaves), stimulation current
- For improving mobility of the vertebrae:
  Active: gymnastic exercises, stretching, muscle exercises
  Passive: chiropractic therapy, massage

> **Important!**
> Taking painkillers and anti-inflammatory drugs long term can produce serious side effects such as stomach ulcers. These medications should be used right away, in sufficiently high doses, but only short term.

COMPLAINTS OF THE UPPER SPINAL COLUMN

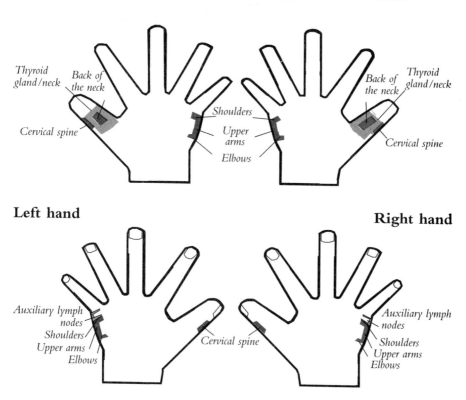

Left hand   Right hand

Main Focus	Left hand		Right hand		Technique
	Palm	Back of hand	Back of hand	Palm	
Cervical spine, shoulders, upper arms, elbows, back of the neck					Energy drainage
——					Energy buildup

5.3 Disorders of the knee joint

Definition

The knee joint is a mechanically complicated joint. The main types of movement are bending and stretching. When the knee is being bent, the head of the shinbone glides past the cylindrical joint surface of the femur. When the knee is straight, the calf cannot be twisted, because this type of movement is prevented by tightened cruciate and lateral ligaments. When the knee is bent, however, the calf can be twisted both to the inside and the outside.

The kneecap also glides over the cylindrical joint surface of the femur. The power of the front thigh muscles is transmitted by means of the kneecap to the front edge of the shinbone. The joint surface of the kneecap, which consists of cartilage, is therefore subjected to great pressure. To the sides of the knee joint, there are two wedge-shaped cartilage disks, the menisci. These help to distribute the pressure from the arched joint cylinders of the femur onto the relatively flat joint surface of the shinbone. If the knee is stretched or twisted too much, the menisci become slightly compressed and may tear.

Common disorders of the knee joint include the following:
- Injuries to the ligaments
- Injuries to the meniscus
- Irritation of the joint through contusions, sprains, or distortion
- Acute inflammation (arthritis)
- Wear and tear, limiting joint function (arthrosis)

Symptoms

Irritation of the knee joint results in:
- Limited mobility
- Swelling
- Formation of an effusion (fluid escapes into the joint cavity)

Meniscus injury brings about:
- Painful restriction of movement

Injury to the ligaments leads to:
- Instability, insecurity, wear and tear

Treatment Guidelines

Acute, inflammatory disorders require these types of treatment:
- Cooling, rest, anti-inflammatory drugs
- Compression (external pressure to limit swelling and effusion)

Chronic, degenerative changes necessitate the following:
- Exercises to maintain flexibility and coordination of muscles

---

Important!
Injuries to the knee often comprise different parts of the knee. They should therefore be examined and treated by a specialist in order to avoid late aftereffects.

120

DISORDERS OF THE KNEE JOINT

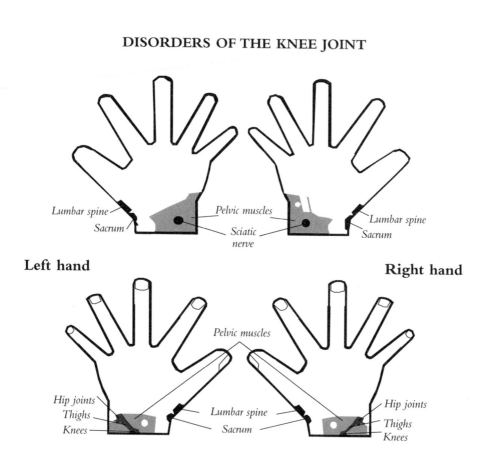

Lumbar spine — Sacrum / Pelvic muscles / Sciatic nerve / Lumbar spine — Sacrum

Left hand

Right hand

Pelvic muscles

Hip joints / Thighs / Knees — Lumbar spine / Sacrum — Hip joints / Thighs / Knees

Main Focus	Left hand		Right hand		Technique
	Palm	Back of hand	Back of hand	Palm	
Hips, thighs, knees					Energy drainage
—					Energy buildup

5.4 Hip complaints

Definition

The hip joints are the links between the upper body and the legs. The spherical shape of the joint ensures a wide range of movements. The head of the femur and the joint socket are covered with a smooth layer of cartilage that ensures that movements are as friction-free as possible. When we are standing or walking, the hip joints have to balance and stabilize the weight of the upper body against the legs. This requires strong muscles between the pelvis, the spine, and the femur. Because of the weight of the body, the hip joints have to bear a great deal of pressure, and constant movement causes an additional mechanical strain.

These are the most common hip complaints:

- Congenital malposition, causing unfavorable weight distribution (dysplasia of the hip joint)
- Premature aging due to wear of the cartilage (arthrosis)
- Painful inflammatory reactions (arthritis)
- Acute injuries (bone fractures, such as fracture of the femoral neck)

Symptoms

Acute inflammatory disorders of the hip joint result in:

- Pain when moving the joint, dependent on the pressure exerted, and in extreme cases even when the joint is kept still

Aging and wear and tear are characterized by:

- Initial pain that improves with further movement

Acute injuries, such as a fracture of the femoral neck, result in:

- An inability to stand or walk, pain if the joint is under strain
- One leg becoming shorter than the other, malposition

Treatment Guidelines

In the case of pain caused by inflammation of the hip joint, the following may be helpful:

- Localized cooling
- Anti-inflammatory drugs (see 5.2, Complaints of the upper spinal column)
- Not putting pressure on the joint, rest

If the pain is caused by wear and tear, different measures are required, such as improving bone and joint nutrition through:

- Becoming gradually more active, doing gymnastic exercises to maintain mobility of the joint
- Losing weight, eating food high in minerals (such as calcium)

In the case of acute injuries or the joint's becoming extremely worn, medicine now offers surgical measures and even a replacement of the joint with an artificial one.

Important!
If you suddenly experience pain in your hip joint without an obvious cause, ask your doctor for an X ray to rule out injury to the bones.

HIP COMPLAINTS

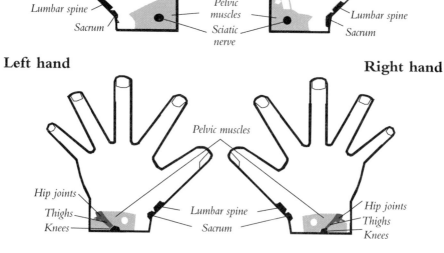

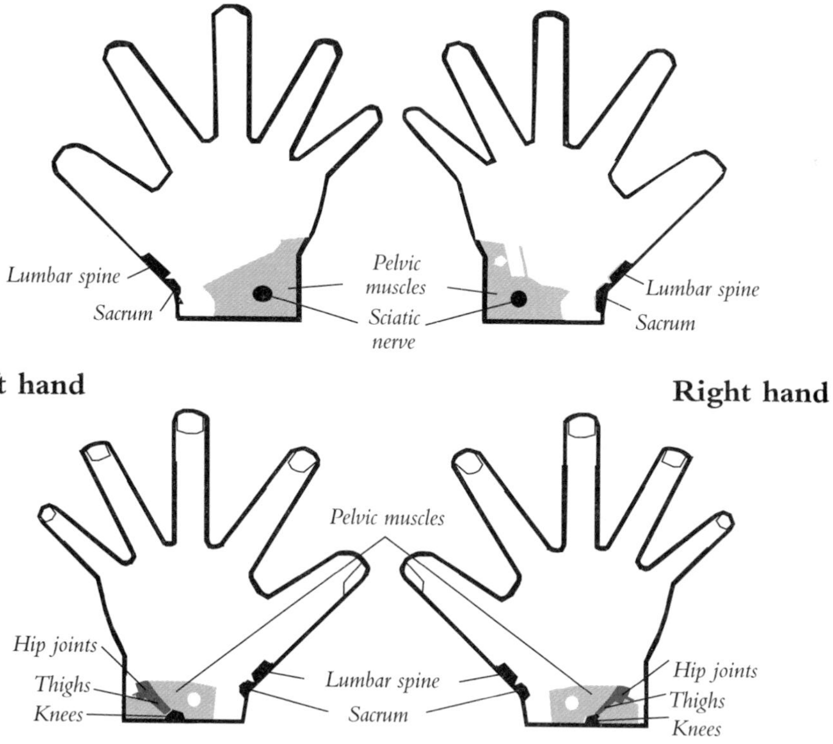

Left hand

Right hand

Left hand diagram labels: Lumbar spine, Sacrum, Pelvic muscles, Sciatic nerve, Lumbar spine, Sacrum

Lower hand diagram labels: Pelvic muscles, Hip joints, Thighs, Knees, Lumbar spine, Sacrum, Hip joints, Thighs, Knees

Main Focus	Left hand		Right hand		Technique
	Palm	Back of hand	Back of hand	Palm	
Hips, thighs, pelvic muscles					Energy drainage
—		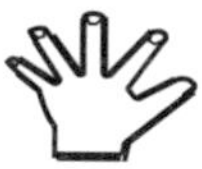	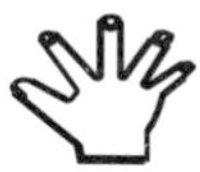		Energy buildup

5.5 Injury aftercare

Definition

The healing of injuries to bones, muscles, and soft parts of the locomotor organs is often accompanied by the formation of scars. Scar tissue is a replacement tissue to fill gaps where normal tissue is missing after an injury, because of inflammation, or due to surgery. However, scar tissue can carry out the function of the missing tissue only partly, if at all. This leads to functional disorders and frequently also to pain. It is therefore important with acute injuries to keep the period of inflammation and the concomitant loss of functioning tissue to a minimum. The interval after an injury is divided into three phases:

- Acute phase
- Healing phase
- Rehabilitation phase

Symptoms

- The acute phase is characterized by the development of inflammation, accompanied by swelling and pain.
- During the healing phase, functional restriction and rest should prevail, allowing scar tissue to form.
- During the rehabilitation phase, when the inflammation has healed, original function is regained.

Treatment Guidelines

During the acute phase, the main goal is to limit inflammation and tissue damage. These are some useful measures:

- Cooling, rest, other means of reducing inflammation

During the healing phase, it is necessary to:

- Close any gaps with scar tissue
- Inhibit inflammatory reactions and alleviate pain

During the rehabilitation phase, the following are beneficial:

- Gymnastic exercises, strengthening of muscles, exercises to improve coordination

---

Important!
Extreme swelling and inflammation can be prevented only through immediate and constant cooling. Frequently, rehabilitation is only successful if pain has been eliminated.

INJURY AFTERCARE

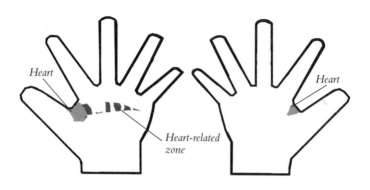

Heart

Heart

Heart-related zone

Left hand

Right hand

Main Focus	Left hand		Right hand		Technique
	Palm	*Back of hand*	*Back of hand*	*Palm*	
Injured body part					Energy drainage
———					Energy buildup

5.6 Muscular disorders

Definition

The term "muscular disorders" comprises a number of very different ailments. Initially, we can separate them into these two categories:
- Ailments of the muscles themselves (injury, inflammation, muscular atrophy)
- Functional disorders of otherwise healthy muscles, as a result of neuropathy, mineral imbalance, diseases of bones and joints

Muscles are made up of fibrous cells whose protein building blocks can be shortened under the influence of nerve impulses. The frequency and the strength of these nerve impulses determine the tension and the degree of shortening of the muscle fibers. A single muscle spans at least one, if not several, joints, and, by being shortened, it causes the joint to bend in a certain direction.

There are always opposing muscle groups at work, enabling joints to be moved into different positions and remain in these positions. The spinal cord controls nerve impulses, so two opposing muscle groups can never be simultaneously activated to their maximum, as this would cause muscles to tear. Such problems arise only if nerve function is impaired, and they are accompanied by pain, tension, and restricted movement.

Symptoms

The most common causes for muscle dysfunction can be found in functional disorders of the nervous system. Typical symptoms include the following:
- Hardening of muscles
- Muscle cramps
- Restricted movement and ability to put pressure on muscles

Acute injuries and resulting complaints are also very common:
- Muscle rupture, contusions, bruises, inflammation, scarring

Congenital or chronic inflammatory muscle diseases are rarer:
- Muscular dystrophy (muscles are poorly developed), muscular atrophy (muscle wasting), inflammation of muscles (myositis, such as in rheumatism), myasthenia (lack of response to stimuli, growing tired quickly)

Treatment Guidelines

In addition to treating the actual causes, muscular pain can be alleviated with the following:
- Cooling, rest, external compressions
- Stretching, gymnastic exercises
- Physiotherapy (heat radiation, stimulation current, iontophoresis)
- Medications to reduce inflammation and alleviate pain (see 5.10, Varicose veins)

Important!
If you suffer from pains in the calves that have no obvious cause, consult your doctor to rule out a deep vein thrombosis of the calf.

MUSCULAR DISORDERS

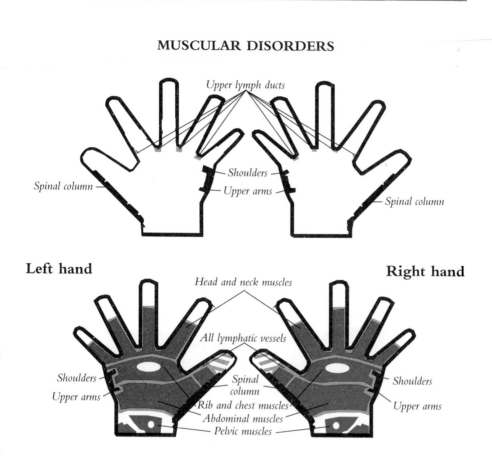

Upper lymph ducts

Shoulders
Upper arms

Spinal column

Spinal column

Left hand

Right hand

Head and neck muscles

All lymphatic vessels

Shoulders

Shoulders

Upper arms

Spinal column

Upper arms

Rib and chest muscles
Abdominal muscles
Pelvic muscles

Main Focus	Left hand		Right hand		Technique
	Palm	Back of hand	Back of hand	Palm	
For muscular pain					Energy drainage
Otherwise, the zone corresponding to the muscle complaint					Energy buildup

5.7 Rheumatic disorders

Definition

Rheumatism (from the Greek for "river" and "flowing pain") is a chronic syndrome characterized by inflammation of various tissues of the body. The joints are most frequently affected, but internal organs can suffer as well. Rheumatic disorders are coupled with the body's immune system, whose main task is to differentiate between foreign substances and the body's own. The immune system is able to recognize toxins and pathogens and to destroy them with an inflammatory reaction. Normally, the immune system cannot act against anything that is part of the body itself. Sometimes, however, this barrier is broken down and the inflammatory defense reaction is suddenly aimed at particular substances in the body, such as joint components, and slowly destroys them. Such autoimmune disorders, in which the body's defenses malfunction and attack the body's own substances, tend to be passed on from one generation to the next, but they can also be caused by an infection with pathogens.

Symptoms

Many different inflammatory disorders fall under the general heading of "rheumatism." Depending on the type of disorder, it can affect all the joints or just individual ones. Common forms and their typical symptoms include the following:
- Bekhterev's disease (stiffening of joints, pain mainly in the morning)
- Polyarthritis (joint stiffness in the morning, attacks of inflammation in the joints, focus on joints in arms and legs, possibility of joint deformation)
- Rheumatic fever (joint inflammation, damage to cardiac valves and kidneys following a streptococci infection)
- Periarthritis (inflammation of the soft tissues near the joints)

Treatment Guidelines

For those rheumatic disorders that progress intermittently, it is necessary to reduce the inflammation as quickly as possible during an acute flare-up:
- Medications:
  Chemical: anti-inflammatory drugs (diclofenac, ibuprofen, piroxicam, corticosteroids)
  Biological: heparin, as ointment, gel, or injection
  Plant-based: horse chestnut, witch hazel, arnica, butcher's broom, echinacea, camphor
- Physical therapies (hot or cold applications)
- Physiotherapy, change of diet, change of climate

> **Important!**
> Effective anti-inflammatory medications always come with side effects. They should be taken only after careful evaluation of their usefulness against accompanying risks. Doctor and patient should be in agreement. It is important to establish the right level of treatment and see it through to the end.

RHEUMATIC DISORDERS

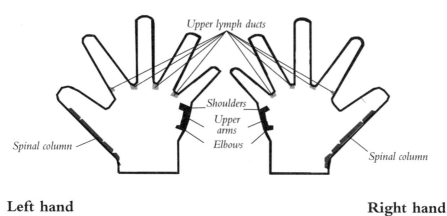

Upper lymph ducts

Shoulders
Upper arms
Elbows

Spinal column

Spinal column

Left hand   **Right hand**

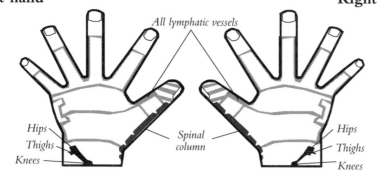

All lymphatic vessels

Hips
Thighs
Knees

Spinal column

Hips
Thighs
Knees

Main Focus	Left hand		Right hand		Technique
	Palm	*Back of hand*	*Back of hand*	*Palm*	
Spinal column, location of disease					Energy drainage
———					Energy buildup

5.8 Shoulder pain

Definition

The shoulder joint is a ball-and-socket joint and capable of a great range of movements. The head of the humerus is loosely supported by its socket, which forms part of the shoulder blade. The shoulder blade is connected to the body only by means of a joint with the collarbone. To the back, its only supports are muscles. The shoulders and arms are served by the brachial plexus, which belongs to the cervical spine.

Shoulder complaints can have their root in the joint itself or in its immediate surroundings. But they often can also be traced back to the cervical spine. These are some common shoulder complaints:

● Wear and tear or inflammation of the joint itself (arthrosis, arthritis)
● Inflammation of the soft tissues surrounding the joint (periarthritis)
● Restriction of movements due to muscular tension
● Complaints of the cervical spine that radiate into the shoulder (cervical syndrome)

Symptoms

The main symptom common to all shoulder complaints is a restriction of movement, accompanied by pain. With inflammatory processes, there are the additional symptoms of swelling and overheating. Severe damage to the brachial plexus may lead to loss of sensation or even paralysis.

Treatment Guidelines

The measures below are advisable for acute inflammatory conditions:
◆ Cooling, rest, anti-inflammatory remedies (see 5.2, Complaints of the upper spinal column)

To alleviate pain and loosen tense muscles, these may be helpful:
◆ Localized heat radiation, stimulation current, neural therapy, wheal therapy

With long-term restriction of movements, try the following:
◆ Stretching, gymnastic exercises, relieving the joint

Important!
Painkillers affect only the way pain is perceived, and they do not remove the cause of the pain. Treatment should therefore include active elements at the start, such as gymnastic exercises or stretching.

SHOULDER PAIN

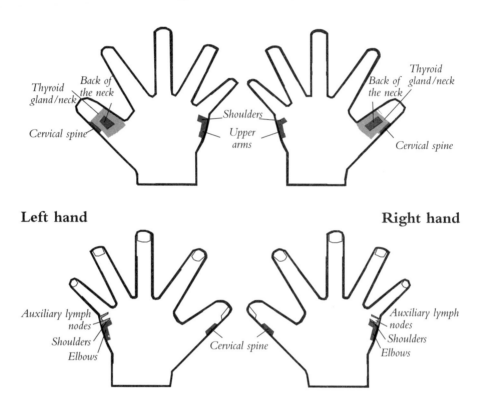

Thyroid gland/neck
Back of the neck
Cervical spine

Shoulders
Upper arms

Thyroid gland/neck
Back of the neck
Cervical spine

Left hand

Right hand

Auxiliary lymph nodes
Shoulders
Elbows

Cervical spine

Auxiliary lymph nodes
Shoulders
Elbows

Main Focus	Left hand		Right hand		Technique
	Palm	*Back of hand*	*Back of hand*	*Palm*	
Cervical spine, shoulders, upper arms, back of the neck					Energy drainage
———					Energy buildup

131

5.9 Tennis elbow

Definition

Tennis elbow (epicondylitis humeroradialis) is not actually a disease of the elbow joint. The name indicates that certain patterns of movement, such as playing tennis, can trigger the condition. It is caused by a stress-induced shortening of the forearm muscles, which are attached to the lateral bulge of the humerus (epicondylus). As a result, even when the arm is at rest, there is still traction on the tendons of the muscles, leading to constant irritation of the highly sensitive periosteum at the point where the muscle tendon joins the bone. Tennis elbow develops as a result of:

- Repetitive strain
- Tensing of the hand when holding something
- Fast, jerky movements of the wrist

Symptoms

These are some typical symptoms of tennis elbow:
- Pain from pressure to the outside of the elbow joint
- Pain on bending the hand toward the forearm
- Pain on making a twisting movement with the forearm
- Pain if the elbow joint is either straightened or bent to its limits

cut 1
line

Treatment Guidelines

During the acute phase, the focus is on pain relief and reduction of the inflammation through:

- Cooling, restraint of the joint, anti-inflammatory treatment (see 5.2, Complaints of the upper spinal column)

In the long term, it is necessary to determine the cause of the condition. Frequently, it can be found in poorly executed sequences of movement, especially if the forearm muscles aren't well developed. The following procedure has seen good results:

- Analysis of the causative actions and thus:
  Avoiding wrong and unnecessary movements
  Correcting technique, especially in sports
  Performing stretching and strengthening exercises for the forearm muscles

Only in a few cases is it necessary to restrain the joint for a period of time—for example, with:

- Tape bandages (keeping part of the affected area steady) and plaster casts

Surgery will lead to only temporary improvements, because the actual causes of the problem are not being removed.

Important!
Strong, compressing bandages can exacerbate the condition. They do not help in avoiding the wrong kinds of movements, nor do they improve the technique of moving the forearm and the wrist.

TENNIS ELBOW

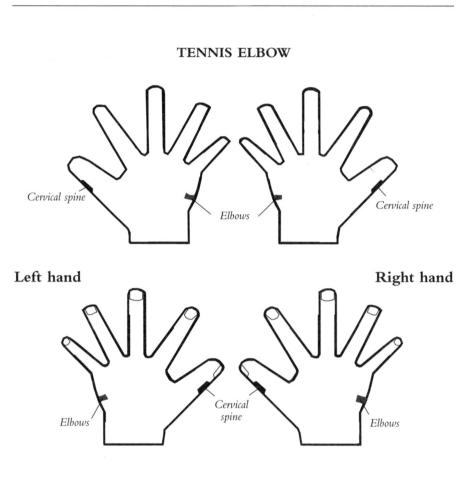

Left hand   **Right hand**

Cervical spine

Elbows

Cervical spine

Elbows

Cervical spine

Elbows

Main Focus	Left hand		Right hand		Technique
	Palm	*Back of hand*	*Back of hand*	*Palm*	
Elbows					Energy drainage
———					Energy buildup

5.10 Varicose veins

Definition

The term "varicose veins" (from the Latin *varix,* meaning "venous node") refers to dilated, winding veins found mainly in the legs. They are caused by:
- Weakness of the surrounding connective tissue
- Defective venous valves
- Increased pressure in the veins

The blood has to flow from the legs against the force of gravity back to the heart. The remaining perfusion pressure is too low to achieve this alone. For this reason, the deep veins of the legs are situated between muscles and are squeezed by alternating muscle tension (muscle pump).

Back-flow valves ensure that the blood flows toward the heart. Should these valves no longer close properly, blood flows back into the lower sections of the vein. If the surrounding connective tissue and muscles cannot absorb the pressure, the walls of the vein become stretched and the vein expands, causing the typical appearance of varicose veins with winding, greatly dilated blood vessels.

Symptoms

These problems are indicative of varicose veins, even though the visible changes characteristic of varicose veins have not yet taken place:
- Swollen ankles, tiredness, legs feeling heavy, calf cramps

Pronounced varicose veins often lead to inflammatory conditions:
- Painful reddening and swelling around the blood vessels
- Formation of blood clots (thrombosis) on the inflamed venous walls

Blood reflux and increased pressure in the tissue result in:
- Impaired metabolism, risk of infection, poor healing of wounds

Treatment Guidelines

The tendency toward developing varicose veins runs in the family to a certain extent. However, the development of this disorder depends on certain factors, so treatment should focus mainly on preventive measures:
- Avoiding sitting and standing for long periods of time
- Walking as exercise to strengthen the connective tissue and activate the muscle pump
- Strengthening of the veins through exercise and physical stimuli (such as water treatments)
- In the case of inflammation, using medicines internally or externally:
  Chemical: anti-inflammatory medications (diclofenac, ibuprofen, piroxicam)
  Biological: heparin, as ointment, gel, or injection
  Plant-based: horse chestnut, witch hazel, arnica, butcher's broom

---

Important!
If thrombosis occurs above the knee, it can cause a pulmonary embolism (a blood clot that has come loose and settles in the lungs).

VARICOSE VEINS

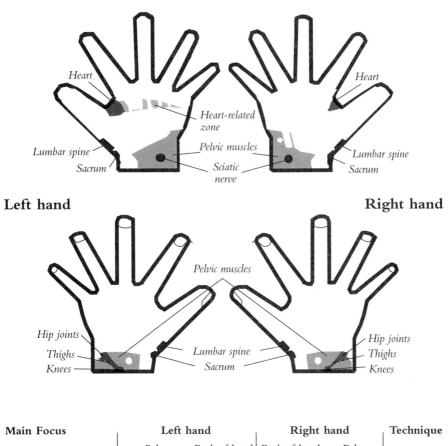

Main Focus	Left hand		Right hand		Technique
	Palm	*Back of hand*	*Back of hand*	*Palm*	
Heart, heart-related zone, hips, thighs, knees					Energy drainage
——					Energy buildup

6. Nervous System

6.1 Dizziness

6.2 Lack of concentration

6.3 Neurasthenia (nervousness)

6.4 Neuritis

6.5 Paralysis

6.6 Stroke

6.1 Dizziness

Definition

Dizziness (or vertigo, from the Latin *vertere,* meaning "turn" and "twist") can have many causes:
- Diseases of the cervical spine
- Changes to the blood vessels that supply the brain, circulatory disorders
- Diseases of the ear (hearing and equilibrium organs)
- Diseases of the brain
- Psychological disorders

In order to function properly, the brain requires undisturbed blood circulation. The two carotid arteries at the front and the two vertebral arteries to the back supply the brain inside the skull with blood. If the cervical vertebrae become damaged, mechanical pressure may be exerted on the vertebral arteries and cause them to narrow. The carotid arteries can become constricted because of deposits or blood clots. The resulting changes in the blood supply will then affect the equilibrium organ and cause dizziness. An unstable circulatory system in which blood pressure is either too high or too low can also cause dizziness. Rarely is dizziness brought on by problems with the brain itself, such as a stroke.

Symptoms

Dizziness is characterized mainly by:
- Unsteadiness when standing or walking, swaying, lack of coordination
- Disturbed hearing and vision
- Headaches

Additional vegetative symptoms occur if dizziness is severe:
- Nausea and vomiting
- Tiredness, exhaustion
- In extreme cases, you can collapse and temporarily lose consciousness.

Treatment Guidelines

If dizziness is caused by changes to the cervical spine, it may help to:
- Loosen muscles, practice stretching, gymnastic exercises, and relaxation techniques
- Take painkillers and anti-inflammatory drugs (see 5.2, Complaints of the upper spinal column)

For circulatory disorders, it's helpful to strengthen the blood vessels by means of the following measures:
- Physical: hydrotherapy
- With medication: hawthorn, gingko, rauwolfia, ergotamines

Constricted blood vessels outside the skull can usually be operated on quite easily. However, the possibilities of treating causes within the skull are limited.

> **Important!**
> In older people, dizziness can be a precursor to a stroke or the result of a serious heart and circulatory disorder.

DIZZINESS

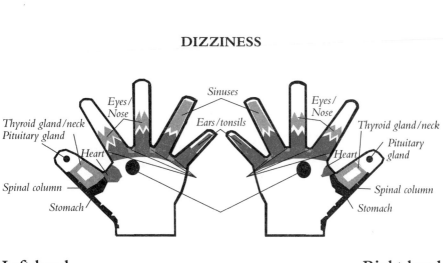

Left hand   **Right hand**

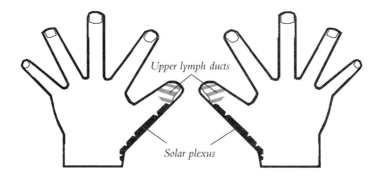

Main Focus	Left hand		Right hand		Technique
	Palm	*Back of hand*	*Back of hand*	*Palm*	
Heart, ears/tonsils					Energy drainage
———					Energy buildup

139

6.2 Lack of concentration

Definition

Concentration means the ability to apply ourselves intensively, purposefully, and effectively to a task. This process comprises several steps:
- Recognizing the problem
- Focusing and collecting our thoughts
- Developing and executing a solution

If just one of the above steps is disturbed in some way, this may make it impossible to concentrate on a problem and deal with it. Such a disturbance is frequently caused by conflicting emotions or inhibitions brought on by emotions. The following factors play an important role in allowing us to concentrate:
- Ability to cope with stress (build up necessary tension, relax)
- Social environment (family, job, position in society)
- Personality (level of education, maturity, experience)

Symptoms

A lack of concentration can manifest itself in many different ways. These are some of the frequent signs:
- Inner restlessness, fidgetiness, undirected urge to keep moving
- Fear, avoidance of conflicts
- Denial, escape into another activity

Frequently, the signs above are accompanied by actual physical symptoms, such as the following:
- Headaches, circulatory problems, nausea, abdominal pain

Treatment Guidelines

As a rule, problems with concentration depend on the individual, making it difficult to give general guidelines. Nevertheless, the measures below can be helpful for nearly everyone:
- Relaxation techniques (visualizations, yoga, muscle relaxation)
- Stress management (making a daily schedule, structuring thought processes and activities)
- Separating formal thought processes and emotions
- Achieving overall fitness (endurance training, mental exercises)

Important!
Sedatives or medications to improve brain performance are not the right way to go when it comes to improving concentration. Their increased use by children has become a problem, actually causing expectations to rise without offering tangible help to solve the existing problem. Medication cannot be used to overcome excessive stimulation (from television, for example), nor can it make up for a lack of physical exercise or counteract problems with the family or the social environment.

LACK OF CONCENTRATION

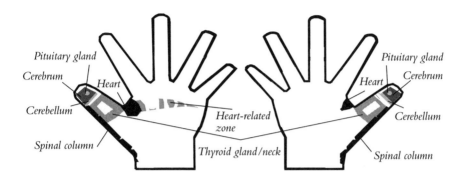

Pituitary gland
Cerebrum
Heart
Cerebellum
Spinal column

Heart-related zone
Thyroid gland/neck

Pituitary gland
Cerebrum
Heart
Cerebellum
Spinal column

Left hand   **Right hand**

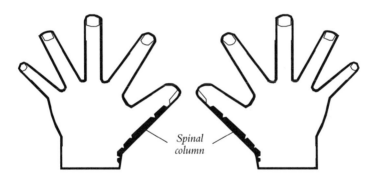

Spinal column

Main Focus	Left hand		Right hand		Technique
	Palm	Back of hand	Back of hand	Palm	
——	🖐	🖐	🖐	🖐	Energy drainage
Brain	🖐	🖐	🖐	🖐	Energy buildup

6.3 Neurasthenia (nervousness)

Definition

Neurasthenia is characterized by the simultaneous occurrence of:
- Excessive psychological excitability
- Rapid exhaustion

This condition mainly affects the emotional levels and the vegetative field (controlling organ function). External influences and internal disorders of the body itself can trigger it. Neurasthenia is frequently caused by:
- Stress, conflicts (at work, in the family, socially)
- Emotional excitement, exaggerated expectations
- Hormonal imbalances (thyroid hyperfunction, menopause)

Symptoms

Psychological signs of neurasthenia include the following:
- Restlessness
- Severe mood swings
- Alternating hyperactivity and exhaustion

Vegetative problems often appear at the same time:
- Undefined pain
- Sleep problems
- Digestive disorders
- Sweating

Treatment Guidelines

It is important for the situation to be analyzed thoroughly, in order to discover the causative factors. Because a person in an acute phase is unlikely to manage this on his or her own, outside help may be necessary if the symptoms are very pronounced. Medication should be used only short-term, as a starting point toward self-recognition and tackling the problem. To this end, the doctor usually prescribes psychotropic drugs with a dampening effect:
- Chemical: benzodiazepines, neuroleptic drugs, antidepressive drugs
- Plant-based: valerian, hops, Saint-John's-wort, kava root, passion flower, melissa

These measures are also helpful:
- Relaxation techniques
- Physical endurance training
- A more conscious lifestyle

> **Important!**
> Psychotropic drugs are highly addictive. Most chemical substances have addictive properties, both physical and psychological, so their use must always be supervised by a doctor. Plant-based remedies are said to cause at least a temporary psychological addiction, but they don't entail physical withdrawal symptoms.

NEURASTHENIA (NERVOUSNESS)

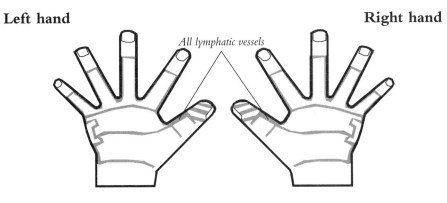

Upper lymph ducts

Pituitary gland
Cerebrum

Heart

Cerebellum

Heart-related
zone

Solar plexus

Left hand

Right hand

Pituitary gland
Cerebrum

Heart

Cerebellum

All lymphatic vessels

Main Focus	Left hand		Right hand		Technique
	Palm	Back of hand	Back of hand	Palm	
Brain, solar plexus					Energy drainage
————					Energy buildup

6.4 Neuritis

Definition

Inflammation of the nerves, or neuritis (from the Greek *neuros,* meaning "nerve," and the Latin *itis,* meaning "inflammation") can be caused by a variety of factors:

- Infection with pathogens
- Toxins
- Dysfunction of the body's defenses (autoimmune processes, see 5.7, Rheumatic disorders)
- Physical irritation

Inflammation of a nerve leads to a functional disorder in the area served by that particular nerve. If the nerve is a sensory nerve, the result can be either a disturbed sensation (paresthesia) or a loss of feeling (anesthesia). In the case of locomotor nerves, paralysis, a lack of coordination, or cramps can occur.

Symptoms

These are the primary symptoms of neuritis:

- Pain
- Paralysis
- Disturbed sensation

Treatment Guidelines

Because the causative factors can rarely be diagnosed, treatment is usually limited to alleviating the symptoms. Pain relief and a reduction of the inflammation can be achieved with:

- Medicines: paracetamol, acetylsalicylic acid, novaminsulfon, tramadole, diclofenac, piroxicam, heparin
- Physical treatment: cooling
- Alternative therapies: acupuncture, relaxation techniques, reflexology

In the case of paralysis and disturbed sensation, the following can be used:

- Electrostimulation (hydroelectric baths, stimulation current), physiotherapy

---

Important!
Suddenly occurring paralysis, a disturbed sensation, or functional disorders of the sensory organs and memory can also be caused by a stroke. If these symptoms are accompanied by a headache, a doctor should check in case of a brain hemorrhage. Functional disorders of the nerves should always be treated by a doctor. The earlier the treatment begins, the greater the chances are of healing or reducing the risk of permanent damage.

NEURITIS

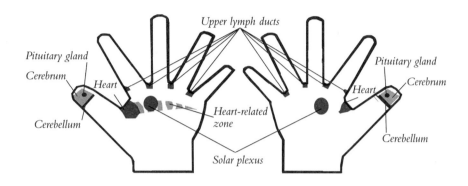

Upper lymph ducts

Pituitary gland
Cerebrum
Heart
Cerebellum
Heart-related zone
Solar plexus
Pituitary gland
Cerebrum
Heart
Cerebellum

Left hand   **Right hand**

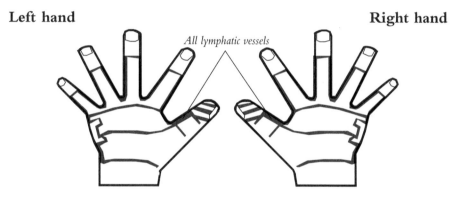

All lymphatic vessels

Main Focus	Left hand		Right hand		Technique
	Palm	Back of hand	Back of hand	Palm	
All lymphatic vessels, heart, solar plexus					Energy drainage
——					Energy buildup

6.5 Paralysis

Definition

Paralysis (from the Greek *paresis,* meaning "becoming limp") develops as the result of damage to nerves that control muscles. The problem can lie with:
- The brain or the spinal cord
- Nerves connecting the spinal cord and muscles

Both usually result in:
- The affected muscles becoming limp
- Increased activity of the opposing muscles, as the control mechanism that keeps these muscle groups in check has disappeared

Nerves can become paralyzed for many reasons:
- Direct injury
- Lack of oxygen in the nerve tissue
- Temporary damage as a result of inflammation or pressure
- Functional disorders due to toxins (such as anesthetics)

Symptoms

The area that the affected nerve usually serves is characterized by:
- Limp muscles
- Inability to execute certain movements
- Changes of blood circulation and metabolism

Long-term or permanent damage can cause the following:
- Stiffening of joints
- Wasting of muscles

Treatment Guidelines

In order to effect healing or limit the damage, the cause of the paralysis needs to be eliminated as quickly as possible. Efficient treatment at the start is particularly important with inflammation and damage caused by pressure:
- Anti-inflammatory drugs (diclofenac, piroxicam, ibuprofen)
- Reduction of swelling (corticosteroids)
- Vitamins that benefit the nerves (B1, B6, B12)

Nerve cells that have died as a result of injury or severe damage are unable to regenerate. In order to improve, you will have to utilize reserves and learn new patterns of movement. This can be achieved with:
- Physiotherapy, stimulation currents, reflexology

Important!
Paralysis is a serious functional disorder of the nervous system, and its significance is difficult for the layperson to assess properly. Treatment should always begin as soon as possible, because the risk of permanent damage increases over time.

PARALYSIS

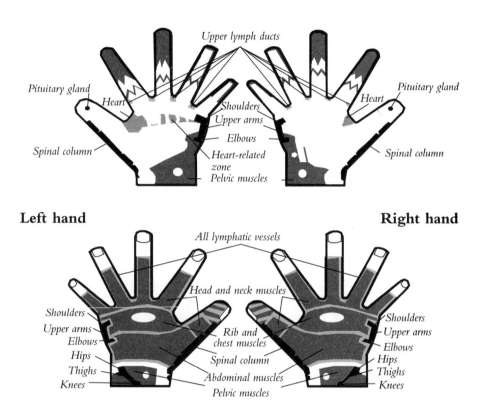

Upper lymph ducts

Pituitary gland

Heart

Shoulders
Upper arms
Elbows
Heart-related
zone
Pelvic muscles

Spinal column

Pituitary gland

Heart

Spinal column

Left hand

Right hand

All lymphatic vessels

Head and neck muscles

Shoulders
Upper arms
Elbows
Hips
Thighs
Knees

Rib and
chest muscles

Spinal column

Abdominal muscles

Pelvic muscles

Shoulders
Upper arms
Elbows
Hips
Thighs
Knees

Main Focus	Left hand		Right hand		Technique
	Palm	*Back of hand*	*Back of hand*	*Palm*	
———					Energy drainage
All lymphatic vessels, all muscles					Energy buildup

147

6.6 Stroke

Definition

A stroke (from the Greek *apoplex,* meaning "slaying") is caused by an acute lack of oxygen in the brain, often as a result of impaired blood circulation. Brain cells react in a highly sensitive manner to reduced oxygen, and, if the circulatory problems persist for a period of time, these cells will die. Because brain cells are not able to regenerate, a loss of brain cells is always accompanied by a loss of brain function. The brain has reserves to compensate for minor, limited damage, but a major loss of cells results in permanent harm. Impaired blood circulation may be caused by:

- Changes to the blood vessels that supply the brain
- Heart and circulatory problems
- Blood-clotting disorders
- Increased intracranial pressure as a result of swelling due to injury or bleeding

Symptoms

An impaired blood supply to the brain commonly causes these symptoms:

- Dizziness
- Headaches
- Temporary loss of consciousness, disorientation
- Speech and hearing impediments, memory disturbances
- Paralysis, loss of sensation

Treatment Guidelines

In order for treatment to be effective, it is paramount for the cause of the circulatory disorder to be diagnosed properly. Initially, it is important to rule out:

- Arrhythmia, vascular obliteration (blocking of blood vessels), thickening of the blood

It is just as important to reduce certain risk factors:

- Diabetes, high blood pressure, raised blood-fat levels, excess weight

Constricted blood vessels located outside the cranial cavity can be treated surgically fairly easily. Changes to the blood vessels generally can be remedied with medications that improve circulation:

- Chemical: pentoxifylline, naftidrofuryl, dihydroergotoxin, nimodipine, piracetame
- Plant-based: gingko, hawthorn, silverweed cinquefoil

In order to maintain brain performance and to activate parts of the brain that are currently unused, it is helpful to:

- Exercise the memory and retention, cultivate intellectual interests and hobbies

---

Important!
Treatment must begin early if there is any suspicion that you have suffered a stroke. Strokes become increasingly likely the older we get, and they are acutely life-threatening.

STROKE

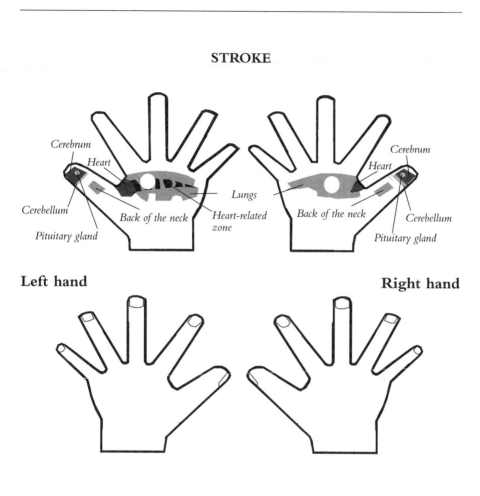

Left hand   **Right hand**

Main Focus	Left hand		Right hand		Technique
	Palm	*Back of hand*	*Back of hand*	*Palm*	
Brain, heart					Energy drainage
———					Energy buildup

149

7. Skin

7.1 Eczema

7.2 Itching

7.3 Nettle rash

7.4 Neurodermatitis

7.5 Psoriasis

7.1 Eczema

Definition

The term "eczema" refers to various skin conditions that are similar in appearance but have different causes. They all have an inflammatory reaction of the skin in common, and can often become chronic. Some of the most common types of eczema, with their causes, are listed below:

- Atopic eczema (neurodermatitis)—due to a general tendency toward developing allergies
- Seborrheic eczema—loose skin scales, as a result of excess grease production
- Microbial eczema—inflammation, due to infection with bacteria or fungi
- Contact eczema—localized allergy, on contact with certain substances
- Dyshydrotic eczema—due to either overly moist or dry skin

Symptoms

An entire section has been devoted to the condition of neurodermatitis. The other forms of eczema have the following characteristics:

Seborrheic eczema:

- Appears mainly on hairy areas of the skin, the back, and the chest
- Characterized by a greasy, scaly, and itchy rash, often accompanied by inflamed pustules

Microbial eczema:

- Ring-shaped rashes, mainly on the arms and the legs and especially in skin creases where moisture gathers

Contact eczema:

- Visible contact area, severe reddening and itching, often on contact with metals (copper, nickel, chrome), detergents, cosmetics

Dyshydrotic eczema:

- Skin that is initially too moist and later dries out and chaps, often on the palms of the hands or the soles of the feet

Treatment Guidelines

Treatment depends on the cause and the stage (acute or chronic) of the condition. Depending on both, observe the guidelines below:

- If the eczema is infected, the appropriate remedies must be used to cure the infection.
- Contact allergens must be avoided.
- Severely inflammatory and allergic forms improve quickly if corticosteroids are used locally for a short time.
- Chronic forms benefit from the use of moisturizing ointments and creams.

Important!
In its acute phase, eczema needs to be treated quickly and effectively. In order to achieve this, topical corticosteroids are often indispensable. Dosage and duration of steroid treatment must be supervised by a doctor.

ECZEMA

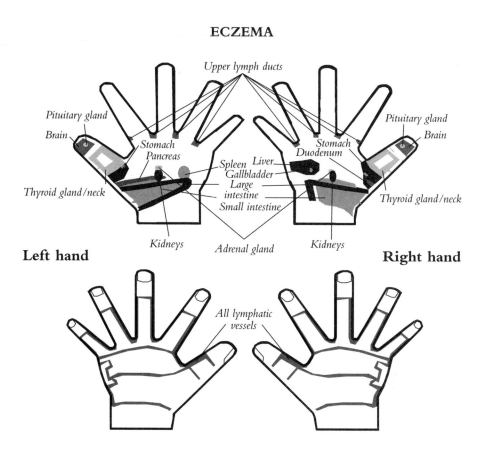

Upper lymph ducts

Pituitary gland
Brain
Stomach
Pancreas
Spleen Liver
Gallbladder
Large intestine
Small intestine
Thyroid gland/neck
Kidneys
Adrenal gland

Left hand

Pituitary gland
Brain
Stomach
Duodenum
Thyroid gland/neck
Kidneys

Right hand

All lymphatic vessels

Main Focus	Left hand		Right hand		Technique
	Palm	Back of hand	Back of hand	Palm	
Cerebrum, pituitary gland, thyroid gland, adrenal gland, all lymphatic vessels					Energy drainage
———					Energy buildup

153

7.2 Itching

Definition

Itching (or pruritus, from the Latin *prurio*) is not a disease in itself but a symptom that can accompany many different illnesses or conditions:
- Very dry, chapped skin
- Allergic reactions (see 7.4, Neurodermatitis, 7.1, [Contact] Eczema)
- Skin infested with parasites, bacteria, or fungi
- Organ disorders (liver disorders, tumors, kidney dysfunction)
- Hormonal changes (pregnancy, menopause, thyroid dysfunction)
- Infectious diseases in general (virus infections, scarlet fever, fungal infections of the intestine)

Symptoms

In addition to inflammatory reactions, histamine-releasing cells often become activated. Histamine is an adrenaline-related communicating substance present in allergic reactions. Besides the itching, there may be an occurrence of the following:
- Stress system becoming activated, causing irritability
- Restlessness, disturbed sleep
- Injuries to the skin brought about by scratching
- Additional infections with pathogens

Treatment Guidelines

If the cause is known, this is where the treatment should begin. However, the causative factors are not always evident. Nevertheless, there are some general treatment guidelines:
- Avoid drying out your skin with aggressive cleansers and frequent hot showers or baths, and care for your skin regularly.
- Target parasites and pathogens.
- Avoid toxins if you suffer from a liver disorder.
Drink plenty of fluids, especially if you suffer from a kidney weakness.
- Relieve itching:
  Internally: antihistamine preparations
  Externally: baths and creams containing tannin, moisturizing ointments and creams, cortisone preparations, antimicrobial combination preparations, ointments with active ingredients similar to cortisone (bufexamac)

Important!
Itching should be treated as early as possible. Scratching causes the healing wound to become inflamed, which in turn causes more itching. If itching is severe and distressing, corticosteroids can be used internally for a short time.

ITCHING

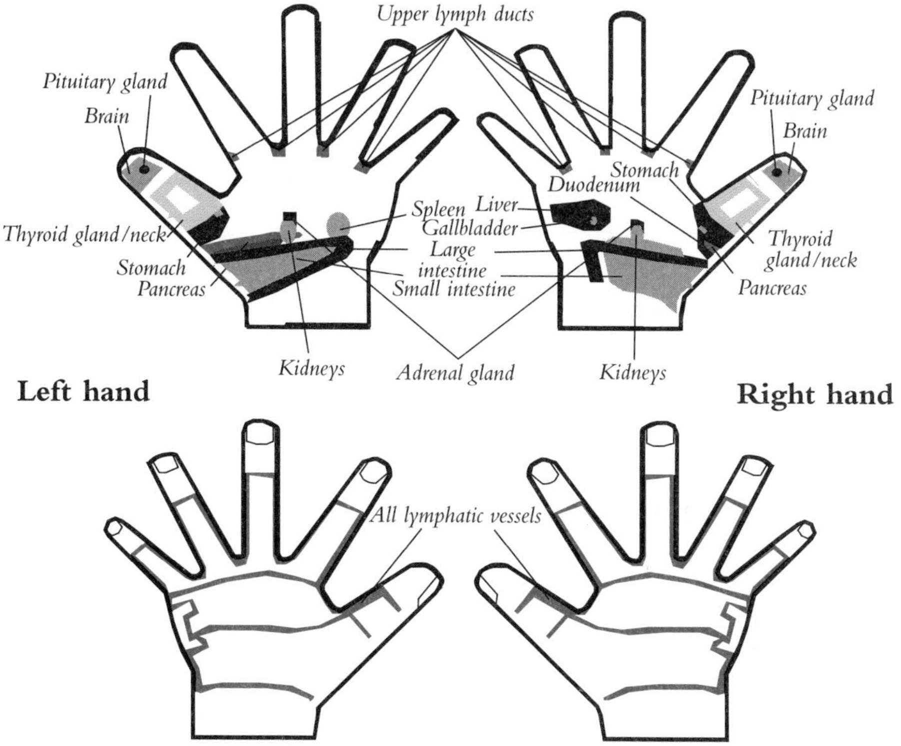

Upper lymph ducts

Pituitary gland
Brain
Thyroid gland/neck
Stomach
Pancreas

Kidneys

Spleen · Liver
Gallbladder
Large intestine
Small intestine

Stomach
Duodenum

Pituitary gland
Brain
Thyroid gland/neck
Pancreas

Kidneys

Left hand

Adrenal gland

Right hand

All lymphatic vessels

Main Focus	Left hand		Right hand		Technique
	Palm	Back of hand	Back of hand	Palm	
Pancreas, thyroid gland, all lymphatic vessels	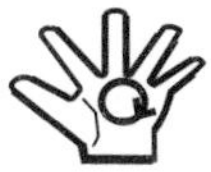	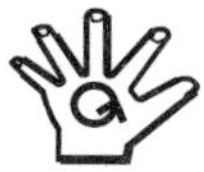	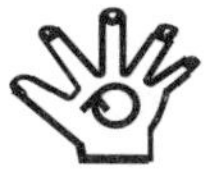	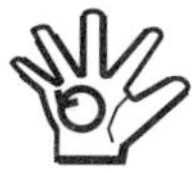	Energy drainage
———	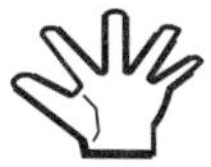	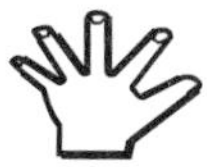	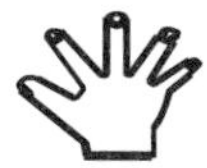	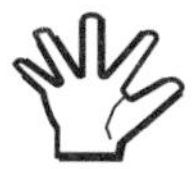	Energy buildup

155

7.3 Nettle rash

Definition

Nettle rash (urticaria, from the Latin *urtica,* meaning "stinging nettle") is characterized by a temporary formation of wheals on seemingly healthy skin. Wheals are swellings on the surface of the skin that develop as a result of fluid collecting in the skin. At the same time, the body's allergy system is activated. Wheal formation is usually accompanied by severe itching and can be caused by a number of factors:

- Mechanical skin irritation (pressure, chafing, rubbing)
- Food
- Chemical irritants
- Medications
- Waste products from bacteria, fungi, or parasites
- Being overexcited or agitated emotionally

Symptoms

- Wheals appear suddenly and unexpectedly, and disappear again after a certain period of time.
- There are no visible changes to the skin before and after.
- If itching is severe, scratching may leave marks.
- During an acute attack, irritation of the skin anywhere on the body can cause additional wheals to form.
- There is a psychological factor, as wheals often appear during stressful times (such as during exams).

Treatment Guidelines

Wheals in themselves do not pose an acute risk. However, their sudden and often extensive appearance can be extremely distressing for the individual. The following points are important:

- Search for a focus of infection somewhere in the body.
- Analyze the circumstances that could have triggered the situation: food intake, psychological stress.
- Determine the cause by trying out different diets or by directly provoking an attack.
- Do relaxation techniques and deal with conflicts and fear if a psychological element is present.
- Antihistamines and corticosteroids are helpful during the acute phase (see 7.2, Itching).

Important!
It is often difficult to determine the exact cause of nettle rash, making preventive treatment usually impossible. Relaxation techniques, reflexology, and visualization can help you to cope better with the situation during the acute phase.

NETTLE RASH

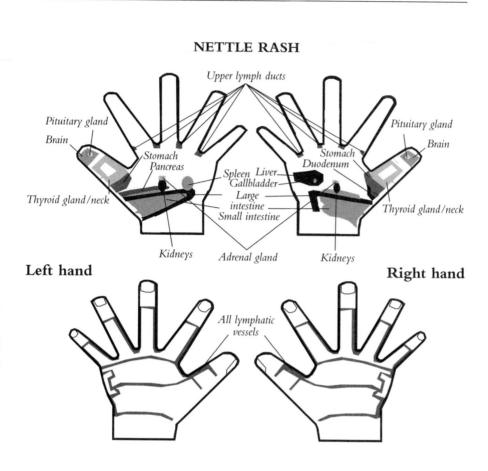

Upper lymph ducts

Pituitary gland

Brain

Stomach
Pancreas

Spleen Liver
Gallbladder

Large
intestine
Small intestine

Thyroid gland/neck

Kidneys

Adrenal gland

Stomach
Duodenum

Pituitary gland

Brain

Thyroid gland/neck

Kidneys

Left hand

Right hand

All lymphatic
vessels

Main Focus	Left hand		Right hand		Technique
	Palm	*Back of hand*	*Back of hand*	*Palm*	
Stomach, pituitary gland, thyroid gland, adrenal gland, all lymphatic vessels					Energy drainage
———					Energy buildup

7.4 Neurodermatitis

Definition

Neurodermatitis is a common form of eczema (see 7.1). It is an allergic condition that, as with asthma (see 2.3) and hay fever, is referred to as an "atopic disease." Neurodermatitis is an inherited condition that often develops in early childhood and usually remains throughout one's life. It can be caused by a variety of factors:

- Allergens (dust mites, medications, food, cosmetics)
- Climatic irritation, change of seasons (spring, winter)
- Environmental influences (air pollution)
- Emotional factors (stress, conflicts, fears)

Symptoms

Similar to eczema, neurodermatitis displays the following:
- Inflamed, itching, reddened skin patches

These skin changes appear mainly on:
- The outside of the knee and elbow joints
- Scalp and hairline
- Hands

Neurodermatitis often occurs in conjunction with other disorders:
- Hay fever and asthma
- Purulent skin patches (furuncle)

Treatment Guidelines

Because it is possible that neurodermatitis is caused by a number of factors all at once, its treatment should cover a wide range of options right from the start:

- Avoiding trigger substances (certain foods, dust, and so forth)
- Undergoing an intensive skin care regime
- Beginning early treatment with medications that inhibit allergic and inflammatory reactions (see 7.1, Eczema, 7.2, Itching)
- Restoring mental stability (relaxation techniques, stress management, coping with conflicts)
- Undergoing stimulation therapies (climatic change, removal of waste products from the body, autohemotherapy, UV radiation)

Important!
Short-term, intensive treatment with highly effective medications such as cortisone ointments is less harmful than ongoing, irregular, and incomplete treatment.

NEURODERMATITIS

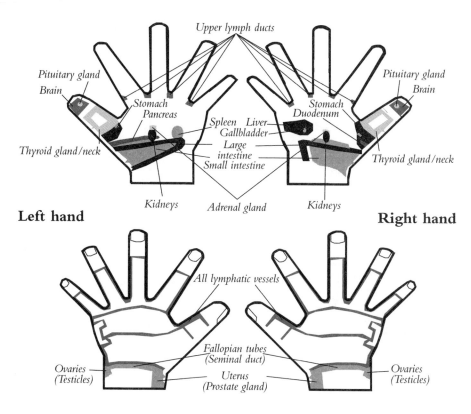

Left hand **Right hand**

Main Focus	Left hand		Right hand		Technique
	Palm	*Back of hand*	*Back of hand*	*Palm*	
Cerebrum, pituitary gland, thyroid gland, adrenal gland, all lymphatic vessels					Energy drainage
———					Energy buildup

7.5 Psoriasis

Definition

Psoriasis (from the Greek *psora*) is a common skin disorder. The tendency to develop the condition is inherited, but the disorder itself is triggered by outside factors such as emotional problems or environmental influences. It is caused by excessive horn formation on the skin, as cell renewal can take place at 10 times the normal rate. Psoriasis usually progresses intermittently, and, in addition to the skin, it can also affect fingernails and toenails as well as the larger joints. In most cases, psoriasis doesn't develop fully until adulthood.

Symptoms

Typical signs are changes to the skin and the nails:
- Clearly defined patches on the skin that are red and scaly
- After the scales have flaked off, thin, very sensitive underlying skin that tends to bleed easily
- Scales forming on the scalp
- Stippling of fingernails (round dents on the nail surface)
- Crumbling nails (crumbling destruction of the body of the nail)

Severe forms of psoriasis can also result in:
- Joints becoming swollen and deformed

Treatment Guidelines

During the acute phase, treatment should comprise the following:
- Descaling with preparations containing salicylic acid
- Reducing the inflammation and normalizing the skin, using preparations containing tar, sulfur, corticosteroids, or plant-based remedies such as calendula, arnica, pansy, violet
- Light therapy
- Climatic change
- Relaxation

Important!

When using ointments, lotions, and baths, it is essential to follow the correct sequence of treatment. Only when the scaly skin layer has been removed can anti-inflammatory and skin-normalizing medications be fully effective.

PSORIASIS

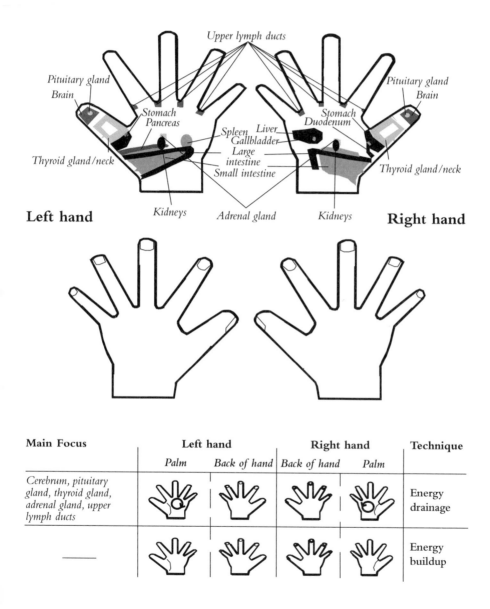

Left hand   **Right hand**

Main Focus	Left hand		Right hand		Technique
	Palm	Back of hand	Back of hand	Palm	
Cerebrum, pituitary gland, thyroid gland, adrenal gland, upper lymph ducts					Energy drainage
———					Energy buildup

8. Complex Clinical Pictures

8.1 Allergies

8.2 Burnout syndrome

8.3 Circulatory disorders

8.4 Circulatory weakness

8.5 Depression

8.6 Diabetes

8.7 Excess weight

8.8 Giving up smoking

8.9 Hypertension

8.10 Migraines

8.11 Pain from scars

8.12 Sleep disorders

8.13 Weakened resistance to infection

8.1 Allergies

Definition

The term "allergy" is often used incorrectly. There is a difference between a mere irritation—for instance, from acids or UV rays—and a true allergy, which is always linked to allergens. These are substances that the body regards as foreign and to which it can display a defensive reaction. Excessive irritation of the immune system due to harmful environmental influences is one of the reasons for the growing incidence of allergies these days.

The following are some common allergens:
- Tree and flower pollen, animal hair
- Foods, preservatives
- Metals, dust, chemicals, dyes and pigments, cleansers
- Medications, cosmetics, personal hygiene products

Symptoms

After the body has come into contact with an allergen, the immune system reacts by activating the inflammatory system, leukocytes, and antibodies. During the allergic reaction, histamine is released. This is a hormone that is related to adrenaline and that triggers the typical symptoms:
- Swelling of the skin and mucous membranes
- Red patches, wheals, blisters, itching
- Stress reaction of the circulatory system (accelerated heartbeat), inner restlessness

Treatment Guidelines

First and foremost, avoid contact with the allergen. If this is not possible, the allergic reaction must be stopped or at least diminished. The intensity of the allergic reaction always depends on the extent of contact with the allergen and the body's tendency toward allergies. If the body itself is under stress, the tendency toward allergies is greatly reduced during the acute phase. During the relaxation phase, however, the tendency toward allergies increases disproportionately. It is therefore important to manage the transition from stress to relaxation as gradually as possible. There are different types of medication available for treatment during the acute phase:
- Antihistamines, which prevent histamine from being released
- Sodiumchromoglycate, which seals the outer layer of the cells that contain histamine
- Corticosteroids, which inhibit inflammatory reactions and prevent dangerous swellings

---

Important!
Reflexology should be used only in mild cases and more as a preventive measure. When it comes to severe allergies in their acute phase, it is no substitute for early treatment with medication.

ALLERGIES

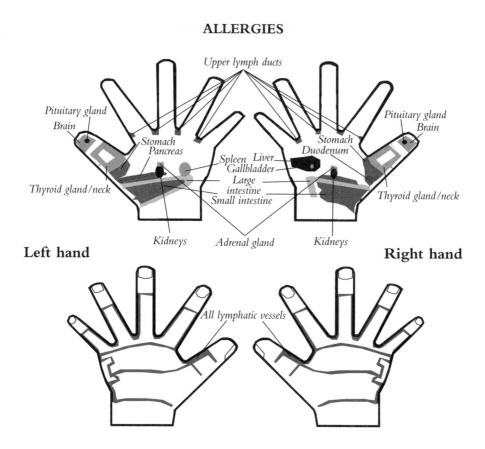

Upper lymph ducts

Pituitary gland
Brain

Stomach
Pancreas

Spleen Liver
Gallbladder

Large
intestine
Small intestine

Stomach
Duodenum

Pituitary gland
Brain

Thyroid gland/neck

Thyroid gland/neck

Kidneys

Adrenal gland

Kidneys

Left hand

Right hand

All lymphatic vessels

Main Focus	Left hand		Right hand		Technique
	Palm	Back of hand	Back of hand	Palm	
Stomach, intestine, all lymphatic vessels					Energy drainage
———					Energy buildup

8.2 Burnout syndrome

Definition

In our hectic and fast-paced world today, more and more people suffer from exhaustion, tiredness, listlessness, and a lack of motivation. For this phenomenon, medicine has adopted the term "burnout syndrome." It affects people from all walks of life. Those who work in the social services seem to be particularly at risk, such as social workers, teachers, nurses, and doctors. It is frequently caused by:

- Constant physical and mental stress
- Working shifts, doing piecework
- Problems at home or at work
- Excessive demands from the environment

Symptoms

The signs below may indicate burnout syndrome:

- Reduced performance levels
- Struggling to meet prolonged, increased expectations
- Loss of motivation and love of life
- Fear of failure, depression
- Isolation and loneliness
- Tendency toward addiction (alcohol, medicines, hard drugs)
- Physical symptoms (stomach pains, circulatory problems, disturbed sleep)
- Physical and mental collapse

Treatment Guidelines

Treatment is most likely to be successful if the initial symptoms are recognized at the start. People need to realize themselves that they are at risk. Frequently, however, warning signals go unnoticed and a collapse becomes inevitable. The following guidelines are useful as preventive measures, during the acute phase, and after a collapse:

- Leading a more aware life (sleep, diet, relaxation, daily routines)
- Relaxation techniques (visualization, progressive muscle relaxation, yoga)
- Time for exercise to release inner tension
- Time for social contacts
- Psychological counseling

Important!
Often people are so caught up in their fixation to achieve that they cannot distance themselves sufficiently from their situation to carry out a self-analysis. In these cases, help is needed from a neutral outsider.

Burnout syndrome is sometimes confused with reactive depression, because the symptoms can be quite similar.

BURNOUT SYNDROME

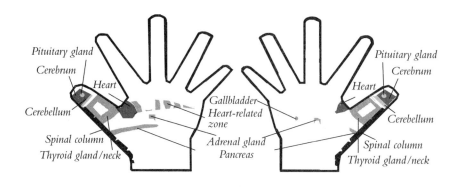

Pituitary gland
Cerebrum
Heart
Cerebellum
Spinal column
Thyroid gland/neck
Gallbladder
Heart-related zone
Adrenal gland
Pancreas
Pituitary gland
Cerebrum
Heart
Cerebellum
Spinal column
Thyroid gland/neck

Left hand　　　　　　　　　　　　　**Right hand**

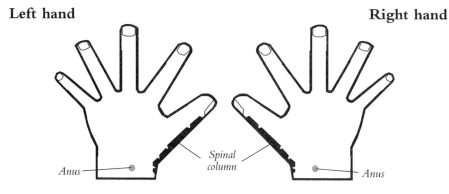

Anus
Spinal column
Anus

Main Focus	Left hand		Right hand		Technique
	Palm	Back of hand	Back of hand	Palm	
———					Energy drainage
Heart, brain					Energy buildup

8.3 Circulatory disorders

Definition

The blood provides the body with oxygen. Nutrients are supplied, and waste products are transported away to the excretory organs. If a circulatory disorder is present, these tasks can no longer be fulfilled where the circulation is disturbed. All parts of the body can be affected, but the following organs are particularly vulnerable:

- The brain and sensory organs (eyes, ears, equilibrium organ)
- Kidneys
- Heart
- Liver

If circulatory problems are severe and persistent, the affected tissue will die and often can only be replaced by scar tissue that is unable to assume the tasks of the original tissue.

Symptoms

Symptoms generally point to the affected organ or body part:

- Brain: dizziness, headaches
- Eyes: impaired vision
- Ears: reduced hearing, ear noises
- Kidneys: kidney weakness, high blood pressure
- Heart: cardiac pain (angina pectoris), weak heart
- Legs: intermittent claudication (cramping pain and weakness in the legs on walking that usually disappears with rest), pain, ulcers, blue discoloration

Treatment Guidelines

Circulatory disorders are generally caused by changes to the blood vessels or by a circulatory weakness. They in turn develop under the influence of certain risk factors. A reduction of risk factors also has a preventive effect:

- Weight reduction to a normal level
- Exercises that benefit the body's circulation
- Normalizing blood pressure
- Adjusting the levels of fat and sugar in the blood
- Avoiding nicotine, alcohol, sugar, and fat

Medications that improve circulation can alleviate symptoms in severe cases. Frequently, however, the changes to the blood vessels are irreversible.

- Medications that improve circulation:
  Chemical: pentoxifylline, naftidrofuryl, dihydroergotoxine, nimodipine
  Plant-based: gingko, hawthorn, silverweed cinquefoil

Important!
Acute blockages of blood vessels cause extreme pain in the affected area, as well as pallor and a loss of function. It's important to seek medical treatment immediately in order to limit any resulting damage.

CIRCULATORY DISORDERS

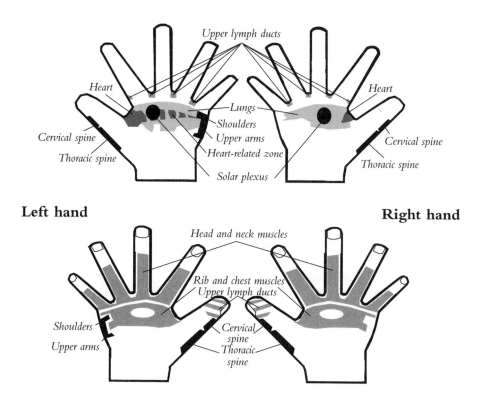

Left hand

Right hand

Main Focus	Left hand		Right hand		Technique
	Palm	Back of hand	Back of hand	Palm	
Heart, heart-related zone, lungs					Energy drainage
					Energy buildup

8.4 Circulatory weakness

Definition

The circulation of blood in the blood vessels is a prerequisite for the body's being supplied with oxygen and nutrients, as well as for redundant waste products' being transported away. The driving force for blood circulation is the heart, which pumps the blood through rhythmic contractions of the muscle wall into the main artery. The elasticity of the blood vessels maintains pressure and passes it on into even the smallest blood vessels, resulting in a pulsating blood flow toward the effector organs. From there, the blood flows back into the venous-collecting vessels and, via the vena cava, is fed back to the heart.

These are some important factors for a well-functioning circulatory system:
- Pumping function of the heart (strength, frequency)
- Tension of the vessel walls (resistance)
- Total amount of blood
- Regulation of blood pressure by the kidneys, adrenal gland, and brain

Symptoms

Circulatory weakness refers to problems relating to the regulation of blood pressure when blood-pressure levels overall are too low. Typical symptoms connected with low blood pressure include the following:
- Nausea in the morning
- Dizziness, walking unsteadily, impaired hearing and vision
- Palpitations and severely accelerated pulse after exertion
- Reduced performance and a general feeling of unwellness

Treatment Guidelines

Low blood pressure doesn't initially present a risk, so treatment with medications is unnecessary in most cases. As an alternative, the following measures may be useful:
- Hydrotherapy
- Gymnastic exercises, activating the muscular pump of the leg to improve blood flow back to the heart
- Endurance training (at least three times a week for 30 to 60 minutes)
- Regular lifestyle (sleeping pattern, diet, relaxation, daily routine)

Medications to raise blood pressure and stabilize the circulatory system should be used only temporarily and in severe cases.
- Medications to stabilize the circulatory system include the following:
  Chemical: etilefrine, dihydroergotamine, caffeine
  Plant-based: hawthorn, ephedra, broom, greater ammi

Important!
Anyone suffering from heart disease must not use medicines that raise blood pressure and stimulate heart function. Many of these preparations constrict the coronary blood vessels and can cause cardiac pain or heart attacks.

CIRCULATORY WEAKNESS

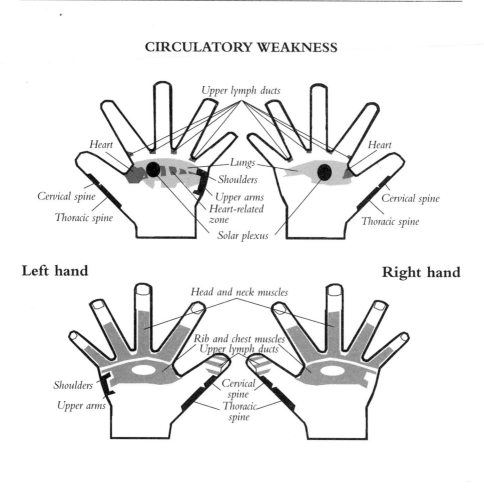

Left hand   **Right hand**

Main Focus	Left hand		Right hand		Technique
	Palm	Back of hand	Back of hand	Palm	
Heart, heart-related zone, lungs, upper lymph ducts					Energy drainage
————					Energy buildup

171

8.5 Depression

Definition

Depression (from the Latin *deprimere,* meaning "to push down") is characterized by the predominance of negative emotions. A wide range of emotions and changes in emotions is part of a full life. Emotions are usually classified as either positive or negative, but there are no clear-cut boundaries, and they are highly individual. Normally, emotions alter from positive to negative and back again in a wavelike pattern. The duration and the depth of the individual phases can differ greatly from phase to phase. With depression, however, there is a definite reduction in the upswing. There are different forms of depression, distinguished by their causes and occurrence:

- Reactive depression, which appears in reaction to a profound experience like a death, a divorce, or illness
- Senile depression, which occurs in old age in connection with involutional processes of the brain
- Seasonal depression, which takes place more frequently during a particular season, such as the dark, cold, and wet time of the year
- Endogenous depression, which is the most difficult form to treat, and occurs without apparent external causes, often also in young people

Symptoms

It's been said that depression has many faces:
- Increasing lack of motivation, lethargy
- Sadness, a predominantly negative view of the world, uniformity of emotions
- Isolation, decrease in social contacts, aggression
- Physiological problems (weight gain, constipation, sleep disorders)

A typical diagnostic symptom is a significant reduction in facial expressions.

Treatment Guidelines

Before treatment begins, the causes of the depression need to be examined thoroughly in order to arrive at an accurate diagnosis. This can be done only by a specialist who will then decide what treatment is best. There are a number of options:

- Psychoanalysis or psychotherapy (especially for reactive depression)
- Stimulation therapy (light, climate, or hydrotherapy, chiefly for seasonal depression)
- Treatment with medications:
  Plant-based: kava roots, Saint-John's-wort
  Chemical: tricyclic antidepressants (mianserin, amitryptiline, lithium)
- General supporting measures (diet, exercise, relaxation)

> **Important!**
> People who suffer from severe depression must always be treated by a specialist. Relatives cannot distance themselves sufficiently from the situation, as they suffer under it as well.

DEPRESSION

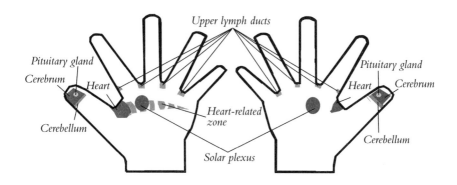

Upper lymph ducts

Pituitary gland
Cerebrum
Heart
Cerebellum
Heart-related zone
Solar plexus

Pituitary gland
Heart
Cerebrum
Cerebellum

Left hand   **Right hand**

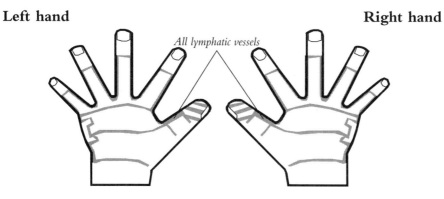

All lymphatic vessels

Main Focus	Left hand		Right hand		Technique
	Palm	Back of hand	Back of hand	Palm	
Brain, heart, solar plexus	🖐	🖐	🖐	🖐	Energy drainage
———	🖐	🖐	🖐	🖐	Energy buildup

8.6 Diabetes

Definition

Diabetes mellitus (in Latin *mellitus* means "sweet as honey") is present if blood-sugar levels exceed 130 mg/dl on an empty stomach. The following two forms are the most common:

- Juvenile diabetes: develops suddenly and affects young people, quickly leads to insulin dependency, is probably caused by a virus infection
- Adult-onset diabetes: develops gradually and affects older, often overweight people, can initially be treated with tablets, tends to be inherited, may be caused by a pattern of overeating

Diabetes develops as a result of a lack of insulin, a hormone that is released by the pancreas into the bloodstream.

Symptoms

A gradual increase in blood-sugar levels does not cause any major problems. Only sudden and severe changes lead to significant reactions:

- When blood sugar is too high: thirst, sweating, accelerated pulse, heavier breathing
- When blood sugar is too low: shivering, cold sweats, racing pulse, tendency to faint suddenly

In addition to the immediate effects produced by changing blood-sugar levels, there is the chance of developing the following accompanying symptoms and subsequent problems:

- Susceptibility to infection and purulent skin conditions
- Itching
- Kidney damage
- Changes to the retina, loss of sight
- Nerve damage and loss of sensation
- Accelerated aging of blood vessels

Treatment Guidelines

With juvenile diabetes, insulin treatment is paramount. For this, there is insulin from animal sources or synthetic insulin, and they are modified to work either slowly or rapidly.

Adult-onset diabetes can be treated with tablets (glibenclamides) that cause insulin to be released from the pancreas. Other medications (arcaboses) delay the digestion and the absorption of carbohydrates from the intestine. Before insulin treatment begins, the following steps need to be taken:

- Weight reduction to a normal level, a controlled diet
- Regular exercise

Important!
Reflexology cannot replace treatment with tablets or insulin.

DIABETES

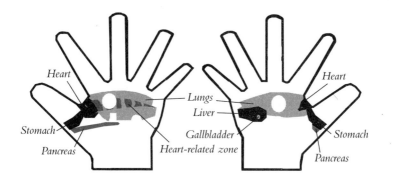

Left hand   **Right hand**

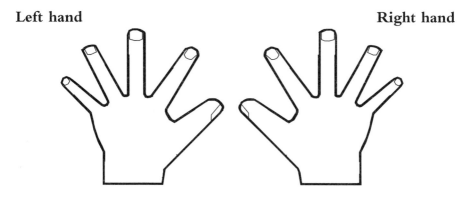

Main Focus	Left hand		Right hand		Technique
	Palm	*Back of hand*	*Back of hand*	*Palm*	
Pancreas					Energy drainage
———					Energy buildup

8.7 Excess weight

Definition

In today's affluent society, an ever-growing number of people are overweight. Excess weight is not merely a matter of appearance, but causes many life-threatening diseases and conditions that diminish the quality of life:

- Heart and circulatory problems (heart attack, weak heart, high blood pressure)
- Diabetes
- Fatty liver, gallstones
- Cancer
- Disorders of the bones and the joints

Excess weight is always caused by supplying the body with more energy than is actually needed. Excess energy is stored in the form of fat. The total daily allowance is made up of a basic requirement and a work-related requirement. Naturally, the work-related requirement depends on the kind of work we perform. For light work, the allowance is set at 30 percent of the basic requirement, for medium work at 50 percent, and for hard work at 70 to 100 percent.

Symptoms

People who are overweight often suffer from:

- Digestive problems (flatulence, constipation)
- Reduced ability to cope with pressure
- Weak connective tissue (tendency to develop hernias and varicose veins)
- Low resistance to infections
- Depressive moods

Treatment Guidelines

It should be easy enough to lose weight:

- Reduce calorie intake (less food)
- Increase energy consumption (more physical labor or exercise)

Yet losing weight means parting with many cherished habits that have often become an integral part of one's life. Therefore, the following guidelines should be helpful:

- Don't follow one-sided diets (they can be pursued only for a short time).
- Avoid eating unnecessarily.
- Avoid alcohol, fatty meats and meat products, cheese, and candy.
- Make time for regular endurance training (three times a week, 30 to 60 minutes of power walking, swimming, cycling, jogging—your pulse rate should reach 140 beats per minute).

Important!
One-sided diets (such as egg diets, bread diets, rice diets, and so forth) are not suited for achieving permanent weight loss. They usually result in only a temporary loss of fluids from the body's tissue. Loss of body fat is possible only through reduced food intake combined with regular endurance exercise.

EXCESS WEIGHT

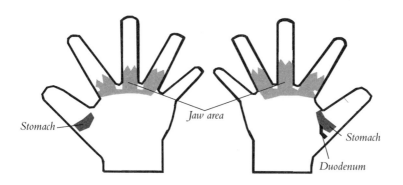

Stomach

Jaw area

Stomach

Duodenum

Left hand   **Right hand**

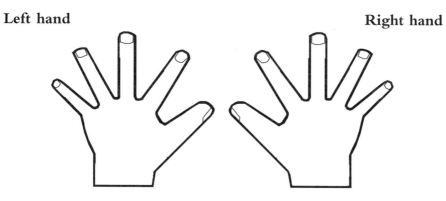

Main Focus	Left hand		Right hand		Technique
	Palm	Back of hand	Back of hand	Palm	
Stomach, duodenum					Energy drainage
———					Energy buildup

8.8 Giving up smoking

Definition

Although smoking used to be regarded as a means of pure enjoyment, for a long time now it has been recognized as one of the leading addictions and a main cause of illness and death. Smokers are three times more likely to die from heart attacks than nonsmokers are, and 40 percent of all incidents of cancer in men could be avoided if these men didn't smoke. In addition, smokers are more likely to develop stomach ulcers, vascular obliteration (blockage of blood vessels), and strokes. In men, smoking is a frequent cause of impotence. Because of the increasing percentage of women among smokers, smoking-related cancers in women are now more common than tumors of the sexual organs. What's more, constant irritation of the respiratory tract results in chronic inflammation, causing premature aging and stiffening of the lungs (see 2.5, Emphysema).

Symptoms

When giving up smoking, changing set behavioral patterns is a decisive psychological aspect. Because smoking is an addiction, stopping the intake of the addictive substance will result in withdrawal symptoms:
- Constant urge to smoke
- Notion of achieving less, discontentment
- Increased appetite
- Restlessness, irritability, depressive feelings

Treatment Guidelines

When giving up smoking, the only aim must be to give it up completely. There is no fail-safe formula for this, but the following factors are important:
- Having positive motivation
- Having unbiased information about the harmful effects of smoking
- Not trying to give up smoking during a stressful period
- Giving up smoking following an illness, when the memories of being physically unwell are still fresh
- Accepting the withdrawal symptoms
- Doing plenty of exercise in the open air
- Avoiding the company of other smokers
- Taking on substitute activities like chewing gum, dried fruit, or carrots
- Banning tobacco from your environment

Important!
If you and your partner both smoke, it's helpful if you try to give it up at the same time.

GIVING UP SMOKING

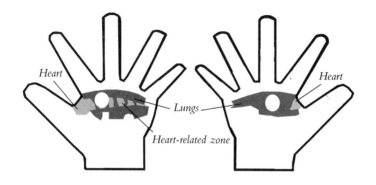

Heart

Heart

Lungs

Heart-related zone

Left hand

Right hand

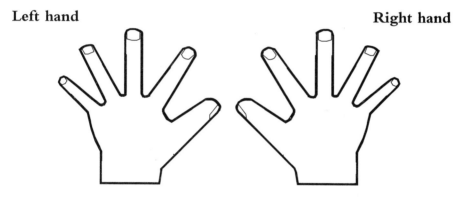

Main Focus	Left hand		Right hand		Technique
	Palm	Back of hand	Back of hand	Palm	
Heart, heart-related zone, lungs					Energy drainage
————					Energy buildup

8.9 Hypertension

Definition

Hypertension (from the Greek *hyper,* meaning "over," and *tonos,* meaning "tension") is the most common chronic illness faced by Americans. The following factors are frequently found to cause pathologically high blood pressure:

- Arteriosclerosis (narrowing and stiffening of the blood vessels due to deposits)
- Stress and tension (increased tension of the blood vessel wall, accelerated heart activity)
- Excess weight and lack of exercise (increased demand on blood circulation, lack of reserves)
- Kidney disease

Symptoms

Raised blood pressure generally doesn't cause any noticeable problems. Doctors are often consulted only when blood pressure peaks have risen to extreme levels and the patient is starting to feel the consequences:

- Breathlessness after exertion or exercise, such as climbing stairs
- Palpitations
- Cardiac pain (see 2.4)
- Headaches, impaired vision, nausea

Treatment Guidelines

If you suspect you may be suffering from high blood pressure, your entire heart and circulatory system needs to be examined. A proper evaluation of the situation is possible only if your blood pressure is checked regularly, both at rest and during exercise. This should be done in conjunction with an ECG and establishing any risk factors. You will not need to take any medications if you have been able to eliminate the causative factors by means of:

- Weight reduction to a normal level
- Reduction of salt intake in the diet
- Regular exercise, incorporating endurance training
- Stress reduction and relaxation exercises
  There are a number of medications for lowering blood pressure:
- Diuretics to increase kidney function (furosemide, triamterene)
- Alpha-blockers to reduce the tension of the vessel walls (doxazosin)
- Beta-blockers to limit heart activity (sotalol, atenolol, propranolol)
- Calcium channel blockers to widen blood vessels (nifedipine, verapamil)
- ACE inhibitors to block kidney hormones that increase blood pressure

---

Important!
All medications that lower blood pressure have side effects, some of them quite unpleasant. They are useful only if they are taken regularly and accompanied by other measures such as weight reduction and exercise.

HYPERTENSION

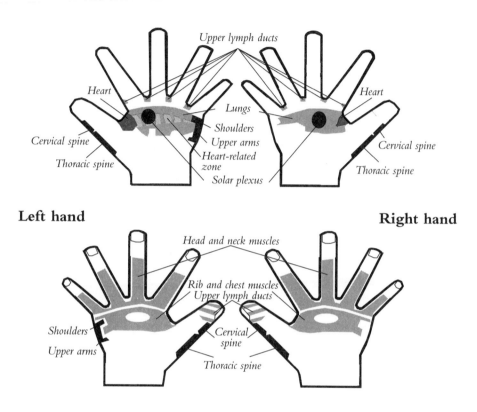

Left hand   **Right hand**

Main Focus	Left hand		Right hand		Technique
	Palm	Back of hand	Back of hand	Palm	
Heart, heart-related zone	![hand]	![hand]	![hand]	![hand]	Energy drainage
————	![hand]	![hand]	![hand]	![hand]	Energy buildup

8.10 Migraines

Definition

A migraine is a particular form of headache that affects a great number of people. It is also referred to as a "vasomotor headache," because an initial convulsion with a subsequent relaxation of the blood vessels of the head has been observed. Next, an inflammatory swelling develops and surrounds the blood vessels, causing a severe headache. The tendency to suffer from migraines runs in families. The actual occurrence of a migraine, however, depends on a number of factors:

- Stress (stress management, handling the transition to relaxation)
- Diet (red wine, chocolate, cheese)
- Lifestyle (sleep, daily routine, exercise)

Migraine patients also often suffer from:

- Circulatory weakness (see 8.4)
- Muscular tension in the shoulders and the back of the neck
- In women, irregular menstrual cycles, menstrual complaints

Symptoms

These are typical signs of a migraine:

- Sudden attack (usually in the morning or on weekends)
- Headache lasting up to several days
- Frequently one-sided, excruciating pain
- Dizziness, impaired vision, light sensitivity, tear secretion
- Nausea, vomiting

Treatment Guidelines

The inherited tendency to suffer from migraines cannot be changed. People therefore have to learn to deal with the condition properly and focus more on prevention than on alleviating the acute pain:

- Avoidance of known triggers
- Regular lifestyle (sufficient sleep and exercise, stress management)
- Natural therapies (water treatments, cupping, autohemotherapy)
- Alternative therapies (reflexology, acupuncture)
- Medications to treat an acute migraine attack:
  Painkillers and anti-inflammatory drugs: acetylsaclicylic acid, paracetamol, diclofenac, naproxen, tramadol
  Vasoconstrictory, migraine-specific medications: ergotamine preparations

---

Important!
People suffering from heart disease must not use vasoconstrictory migraine medications.

Sudden, excruciating headaches should be examined by a neurologist, because they could also signal a brain hemorrhage.

MIGRAINES

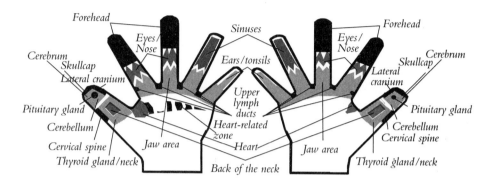

Forehead · Eyes/Nose · Sinuses · Forehead · Eyes/Nose
Cerebrum · Skullcap · Lateral cranium · Ears/tonsils · Cerebrum · Skullcap · Lateral cranium
Pituitary gland · Upper lymph ducts · Pituitary gland
Cerebellum · Heart-related zone · Cerebellum · Cervical spine
Cervical spine · Jaw area · Heart · Jaw area
Thyroid gland/neck · Back of the neck · Thyroid gland/neck

Left hand   **Right hand**

Frontal and maxillary sinuses
Head and neck muscles
Upper lymph ducts
Cervical spine

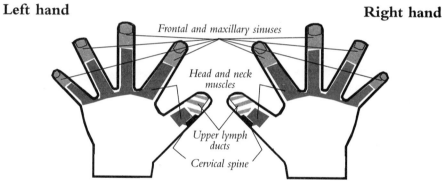

Main Focus	Left hand		Right hand		Technique
	Palm	Back of hand	Back of hand	Palm	
Heart, neck muscles, eyes, nose					Energy drainage
——					Energy buildup

8.11 Pain from scars

Definition

Following an injury or an inflammation, many cells die in the affected area of the body, and the subsequent gaps are filled by scar tissue. But scar tissue is not a fully functioning substitute for the original tissue, such as in muscles, bones, joints, tendons, internal organs, and nerves. Initially, a fresh scar is numb and poorly supplied with blood. With time, however, small blood vessels and nerves find their way into the scar, blood circulation improves, and sensation increases. At first, these sensations are difficult to differentiate and are often perceived as pain. Only with time does the body become familiar with the new nerve signals, and they lose their pain character.

In the case of injuries, often larger nerves are destroyed. Once nerve fibers have been severed, they are usually unable to regenerate, and the remaining functional part of the nerve ends in a scar. There, mechanical irritation still produces nerve signals that the body perceives as coming from the area originally served by this particular nerve. After an amputation, for example, people often report painful sensations from the amputated limb—this is called "phantom limb pain."

Symptoms

These problems often occur when there is scar tissue:
- Loss of sensation
- Increased sensitivity to pain
- Disturbed perception of hot and cold
- Impaired circulation, wound not healing properly

Treatment Guidelines

Depending on the location, the extent, and the age of the scar, different measures are called for:
- Fresh scars: rest, avoiding unnecessary strain on the scar
- Scars with poor blood supply: light massages, alternating hot and cold baths, exercise
- Scars that are not healing properly: surgical removal of the tissue that isn't receiving sufficient blood
- Scars with increased sensitivity: massages, exercises, slowly increasing stimulation
- Painful scars: local anesthetic, severing of nerves outside the scar, increasing stimulation, reflexology, acupuncture

---

Important!
If scars are treated prematurely, this can result in the formation of too much scar tissue and increased sensitivity.

PAIN FROM SCARS

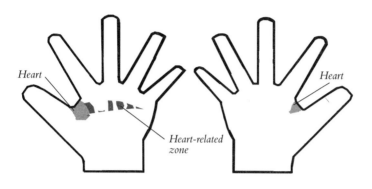

Heart

Heart-related zone

Heart

Left hand

Right hand

Main Focus	Left hand		Right hand		Technique
	Palm	*Back of hand*	*Back of hand*	*Palm*	
Scar area	🖐	🖐	🖐	🖐	Energy drainage
———	🖐	🖐	🖐	🖐	Energy buildup

8.12 Sleep disorders

Definition

Sleep is designed to aid regeneration and help build reserves. During sleeping hours, the body's metabolism changes and available energy can be used for growth and repair processes. But sleep also fulfills an important task for the nervous system and the psyche: All the impressions and emotions from the waking hours are sorted and processed. Tensions brought on from excessive stimulation can be released, and the short-term memory is emptied so that it can deal with new impressions. During the sleep phase, there is an exchange between the conscious and the subconscious, and this manifests itself in dreams where fantasy and reality come together.

As we grow older, we need less and less sleep. Whereas infants sleep for up to 18 hours a day, adults require only about eight hours of sleep and older people often manage with just six. But the quality of our sleep is not determined merely by the number of hours we spend asleep. Alternating phases of sleep (such as REM sleep) and the depth of sleep are important too. Only when all these requirements are met do we experience restful sleep, and can we start the new day feeling well rested, fresh, and full of energy.

Symptoms

Sleep disorders are a common problem today. Internal factors such as illness are rarely the trigger. More often external influences are responsible for troubled sleep:

■ Stress (for instance, because of working night shifts or doing piecework), insufficient relaxation
■ Frequent trips to different time zones
■ Unhealthy lifestyle (poor diet, lack of exercise)
■ Social conflicts (relationship, family)

A lack of sleep causes a greater susceptibility to harmful influences both internally and externally, giving rise to a vicious cycle that constantly reinforces itself.

Treatment Guidelines

The key to a good night's sleep lies in leading a healthy lifestyle:

◆ Relaxation periods throughout the day
◆ Sufficient exercise
◆ Avoiding nicotine, alcohol, drugs
◆ Avoiding excessive stimulation (television, computers, discos)
◆ Sleep-inducing drugs should only be used rarely and over a short period:
  Chemical: benzodiazepine, zolpidem, zopiclon, chloral hydrate
  Plant-based: valerian, hops, Saint-John's-wort, melissa, passion flower

---

Important!
Chemical sleep-inducing drugs cannot improve the quality of sleep. They merely serve as aids for falling asleep, and should be used only short term because of their highly addictive properties.

SLEEP DISORDERS

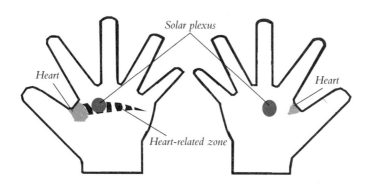

Solar plexus

Heart

Heart

Heart-related zone

Left hand   **Right hand**

Main Focus	Left hand		Right hand		Technique
	Palm	*Back of hand*	*Back of hand*	*Palm*	
Solar plexus					Energy drainage
———					Energy buildup

8.13 Weakened resistance to infection

Definition

Infections with pathogens pose a constant risk to the human body. The immune system is a complicated defensive system and is able to recognize pathogens and foreign substances, rendering them inactive or destroying them. Important components of the immune system include white blood cells (leukocytes), lymphatic organs (lymph nodes, lymphatic vessels, spleen), and special proteins (antibodies or immunoglobulins). In addition to an immediate reaction, the immune system is able to store information about pathogens and can therefore release appropriate leukocytes and antibodies the next time it encounters them. AIDS has made the significance of the immune system very clear, but it isn't just serious diseases such as AIDS or leukemia that affect the immune system. Many people today are increasingly susceptible to infection. The body's defenses work because of an equilibrium of activation and inhibition. However, internal and external stress factors can upset this balance:

- Excess weight, poor diet, alcohol, nicotine
- Stress, lack of sleep
- Pollution (exhaust fumes, smog, dust, pesticides, poisons, chemicals, dyes and pigments)

Symptoms

A weakened resistance to infection manifests itself especially where the body comes into contact with the environment (respiratory system, digestive system, mouth and pharynx, bladder, skin), and it can cause the following:

- Frequent and persistent illnesses of the respiratory tract
- Repeated infections of the urinary tract
- Chronic infections of the digestive tract caused by bacteria or fungi
- Repeated, purulent infections of the skin, persistent fungal infections of the skin

Treatment Guidelines

During an acute infection, therapy depends on the type of pathogen and how dangerous it is. In addition to general advice regarding infectious diseases (rest, increased fluid intake, bed rest if suffering from fever, plenty of sleep), the following measures are useful to boost the immune system:

- Lifestyle (stress reduction, relaxation, healthy diet)
- Exercise (for mobility and endurance)
- Hydrotherapy (cold water treatment, cold compresses and packs)
- Stimulation therapy (climate change, sauna, UV radiation)
- Treatment to stimulate the immune system (autohemotherapy, microbiological therapy)

> **Important!**
> Severe, persistent infections and infections accompanied by a high fever must be treated by a doctor.

WEAKENED RESISTANCE TO INFECTION

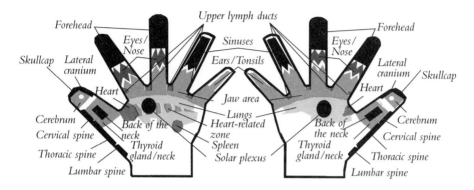

Forehead
Eyes/Nose
Upper lymph ducts
Sinuses
Ears/Tonsils
Forehead
Eyes/Nose
Skullcap
Lateral cranium
Lateral cranium
Skullcap
Heart
Jaw area
Heart
Cerebrum
Cervical spine
Back of the neck
Lungs
Heart-related zone
Spleen
Solar plexus
Back of the neck
Cerebrum
Cervical spine
Thoracic spine
Thyroid gland/neck
Thyroid gland/neck
Thoracic spine
Lumbar spine
Lumbar spine

Left hand **Right hand**

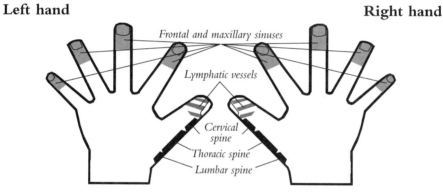

Frontal and maxillary sinuses
Lymphatic vessels
Cervical spine
Thoracic spine
Lumbar spine

Main Focus	Left hand		Right hand		Technique
	Palm	Back of hand	Back of hand	Palm	
Upper lymph ducts, heart, lungs, spleen					Energy drainage
―――					Energy buildup

Index